THE BLOB GUIDE TO
CHILDREN'S HUMAN RIGHTS

This practical resource is designed to support children and young people as they develop an understanding of the basic rights that we are all entitled to as humans. Diverse and inclusive, Blob figures have proven themselves to be a valuable way of sparking discussion of difficult topics through the universal means of body language and feelings.

Based upon the UN Convention on the Rights of the Child, this book introduces 'Blob Trees', lines and images with prompt questions and activities to help children to consider concepts such as freedom of movement and speech, safety and equality. It encourages children to think about the ways in which they can apply human rights articles to their own lives, by treating others with kindness, fairness and respect.

Key features include:

- 'How to use' guides and prompt questions for each topic
- Simplified and child-friendly versions of all 42 human rights articles
- Photocopiable and downloadable worksheets designed to be used with individuals and groups of all sizes.

With clear and supportive guidance and a graduated approach, this is an essential tool for teachers and practitioners looking to support an understanding of human rights in children and young people. It will also be invaluable for any groups wishing to develop accreditation for UNICEF's 'Rights Respecting Schools' Awards.

Pip Wilson is the author of over fifty books and the famous 'Blob Tree' tools, which can open the hardest heart, and is able to open up meaningful communication in all cultures and contexts. His work has ranged from street gangs, Hells Angels, people with drug and alcohol issues, and charity housing projects. He currently works as a freelance people worker, conducting groupwork/training/facilitation in the corporate and voluntary sectors. He believes that there is no such thing as a difficult person – only difficult behaviour.

Ian Long is an illustrator who has worked with Pip all of his adult life, drawing, creating and visualising ideas that they have imagined together since the early 1980s. He has been a youth and pastoral worker in Gloucestershire, a primary school teacher in West Sussex and Hampshire, a carer for his father who suffered with Alzheimer's and is now working full time on books. He is married to Jane, and they have two beautiful adult daughters.

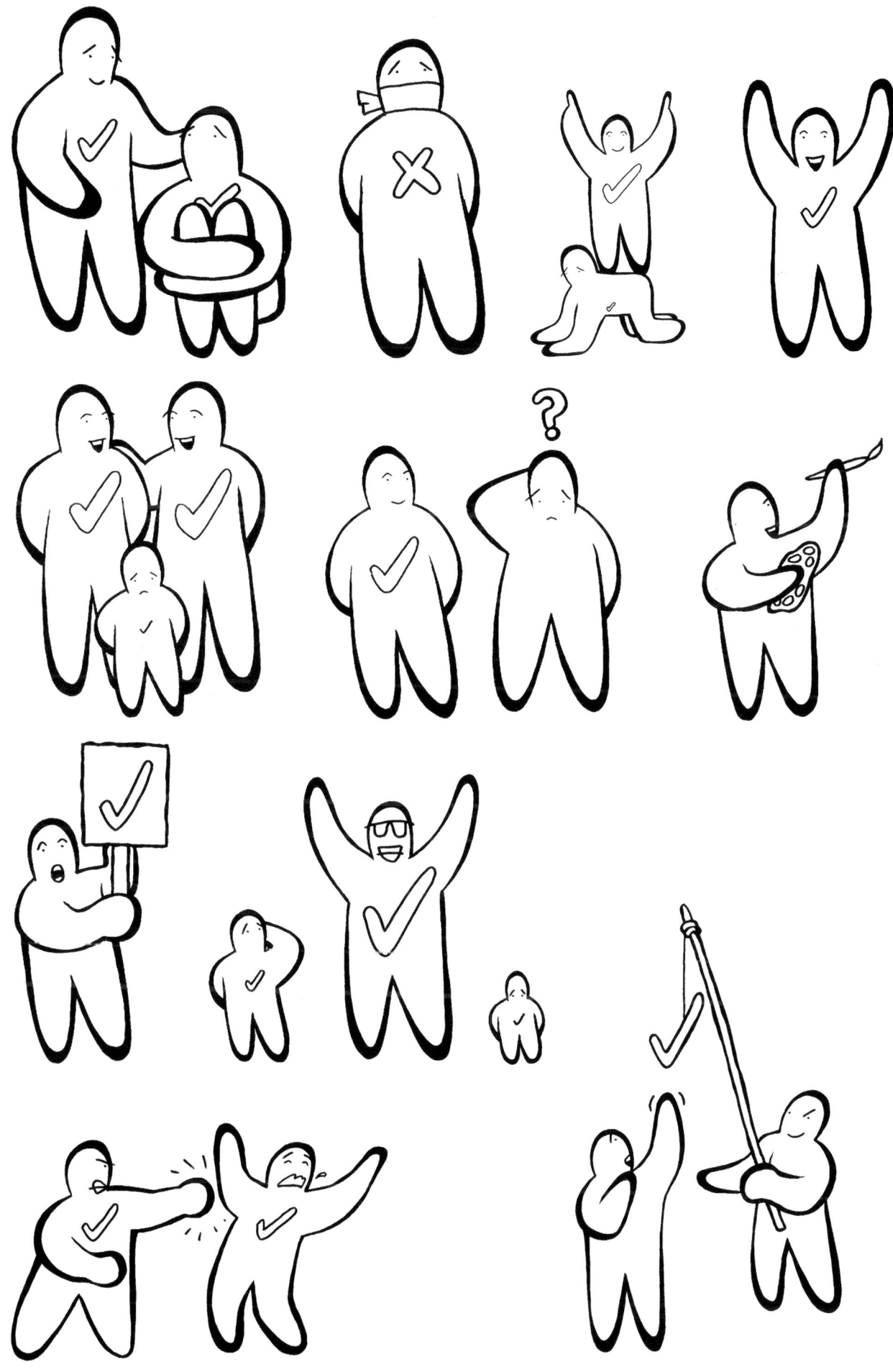

Series URL: www.routledge.com/Blobs/book-series/BLOBS

Blobs

Blobs are delightful characters (without gender or age) that help facilitate and stimulate meaningful discussions about difficult issues or situations. Individuals or groups can start discussions by identifying themselves, or others, with an individual or group of Blobs whose actions or feelings represent their own.

The series includes a range of activities, books and posters, suitable for all ages.

Authors – Pip Wilson and Ian Long

Titles in this series include:

The Blob Guide to Children's Human Rights

The Big Book of Blobs (2nd edition)

The Big Book of Blob Trees (2nd edition)

The Big Book of Blob Feelings

The Big Book of Blob Feelings 2

The Blob Anger Book

Feelings Blob Cards

Emotions Blob Cards

Anger Blob Cards

Bereavement Blob Cards

Behaviour Blob Cards

Family Blob Cards

Teenage Life Blob Cards

Blob School

The Blob Visual Emotional Thesaurus

Giant Blob Tree Poster

Blob Feelings Ball

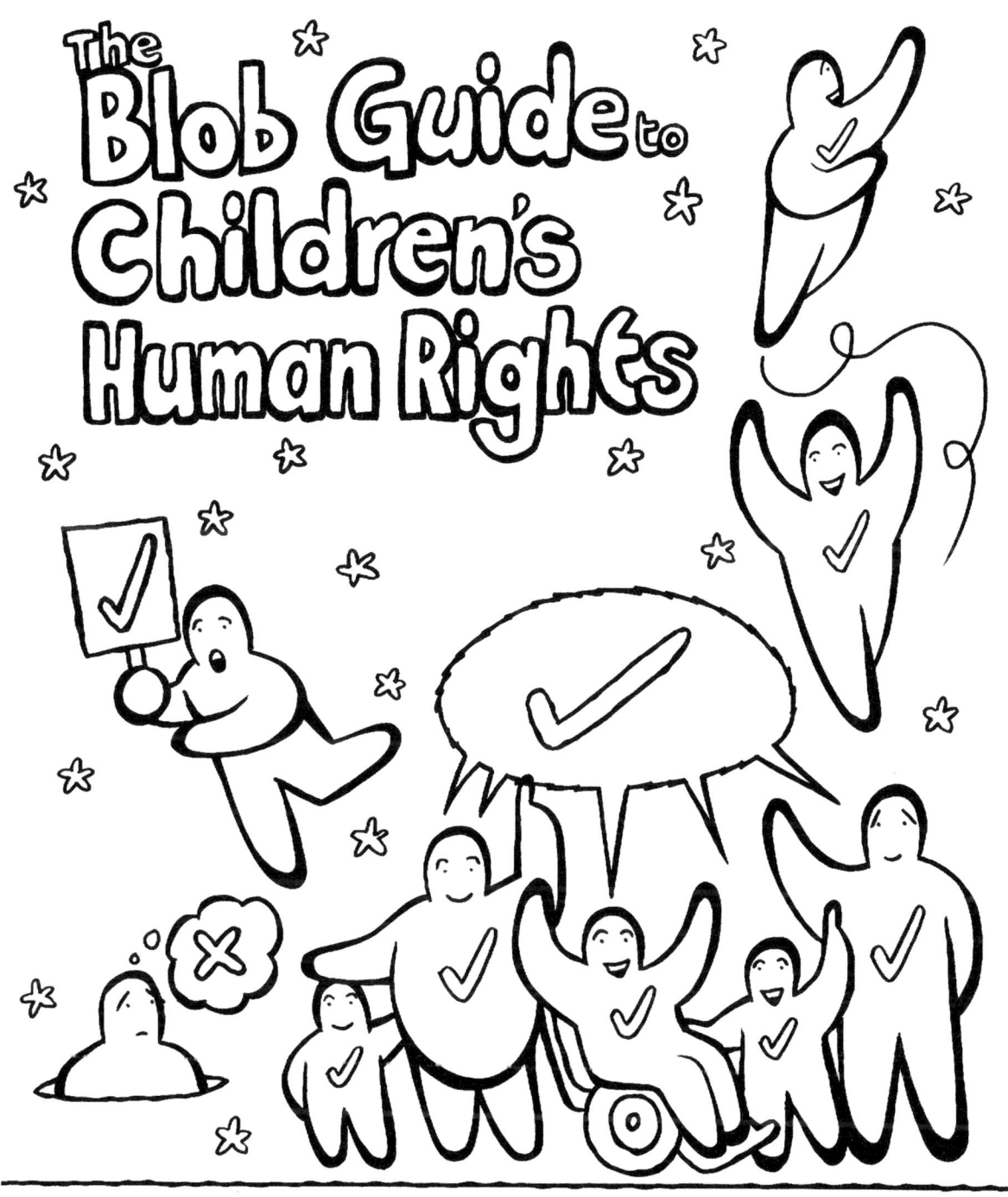

The Blob Guide to Children's Human Rights

Pip Wilson + Ian Long

THE BLOB GUIDE TO

CHILDREN'S HUMAN RIGHTS

Pip Wilson and Ian Long

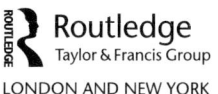
Routledge
Taylor & Francis Group

LONDON AND NEW YORK

THE BLOB GUIDE TO
CHILDREN'S HUMAN RIGHTS

First published 2021
by Routledge
2 Park Square, Milton Park, Abingdon, Oxon OX14 4RN

and by Routledge
52 Vanderbilt Avenue, New York, NY 10017

Routledge is an imprint of the Taylor & Francis Group, an informa business

British Library Cataloguing-in-Publication Data
A catalogue record for this book is available from the British Library

Library of Congress Cataloging-in-Publication Data
Names: Wilson, Pip, author. | Long, Ian, author. | Routledge (Firm)
Title: The blob guide to children's human rights / Pip Wilson and Ian Long.
Description: First Edition. | New York : Routledge, 2020.
Identifiers: LCCN 2020023833 (print) | LCCN 2020023834 (ebook) |
ISBN 9780367561550 (Hardback) | ISBN 9780367561543 (Paperback) |
ISBN 9781003096641 (eBook)
Subjects: LCSH: Imagery (Psychology)–Therapeutic use. |
Children's rights. | Art therapy.
Classification: LCC RC489.F35 W56 2020 (print) |
LCC RC489.F35 (ebook) | DDC 616.89/1656–dc3
LC record available at https://lccn.loc.gov/2020023833
LC ebook record available at https://lccn.loc.gov/2020023834

ISBN: 978-0-367-56155-0 (hbk)
ISBN: 978-0-367-56154-3 (pbk)
ISBN: 978-1-003-09664-1 (ebk)

Typeset in Helvetica
by Newgen Publishing UK

Visit the companion website: www.routledge.com/cw/speechmark

Dedicated to all those whose human rights are denied by oppressive governments around the world

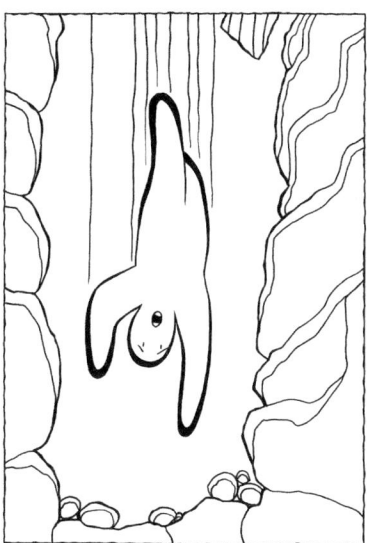

Contents

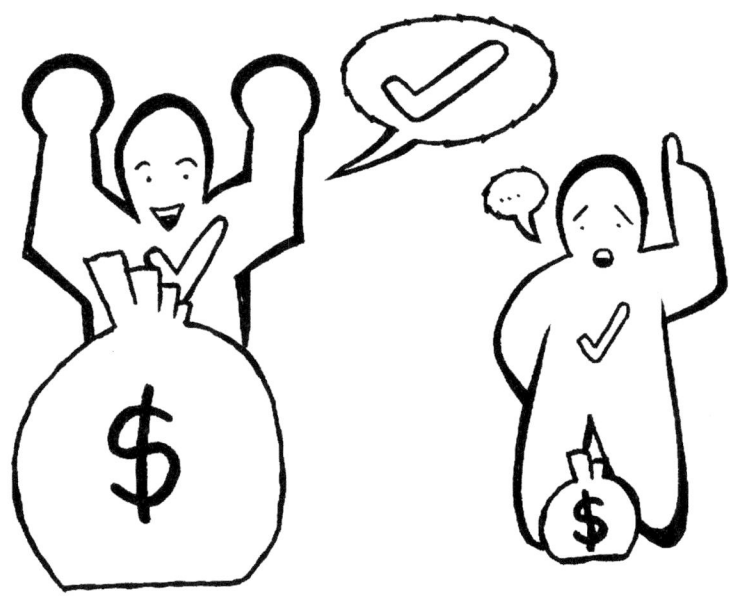

CHILDREN'S HUMAN RIGHTS

Introduction

Human rights are becoming the global measure for a nation's health. In some parts of the world, health and wealth are very important, whereas freedom of movement and religion are denied. In other parts of our globe, these rights are reversed. Each nation prioritises the values that it holds above all the others. This book is an attempt to introduce children to all the aspects of the UN Convention on the Rights of the Child (UNCRC), regardless of their nation's particular preferences. It is based upon the UNICEF children's version.

Some of the topics are more suited to older children whilst others can be adapted for all ages. In the main human rights article section you will find a simplified version of all forty-two rights as imagined by Heathfield School, which we worked with whilst creating these visual tools. The teacher, Mark, and his human rights council were very appreciative of all the tools that we sent in their direction. The more that families become aware of their rights, the more that all of us will support each other's personal growth and sense of worth.

Each section has its own 'how to use' introduction, and a unique approach to the topic. Under the suggested questions for each visual tool, there is space for you to add your own comments. With Ian having been a primary school teacher for seventeen years, making each resource relevant to the group of children with whom he's working is absolutely essential.

We hope that this book will help children and adults to support individuals, schools, families and communities to become more aware of human rights and to grow into a nation that lives out each and every article.

Pip and Ian

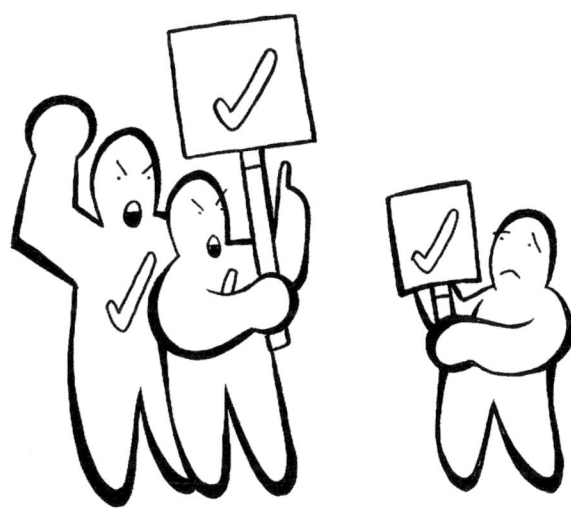

How to Use the Blobs – Blob Feelosophy

Blobs are a way of communicating using two of the first languages that we learn as children – body language and feelings. Before we can speak, before we can write, we have all learned to read the signs in our parents' faces, and appreciate being held and hugged. This means that Blobs are an all-age resource. In Ian's own school work, he has used them with children as young as four who have already begun to recognise when they feel like these 'funny people'. Blobs live in a strange world that our eyes cannot see but our heart can discern. We can learn to 'read' the world emotionally and identify who is walking around with a thundercloud over their lives or is like the sun bursting forth!

We can learn a new way of seeing – emotionally.

Blobs work best when we take the time to start with ourselves. We wouldn't dream of teaching a child to tie their laces if we hadn't learned to do it first ourselves. Likewise, we need to reflect upon our own hearts using Blobs before we encourage others to do the same. Pip and Ian have found that the best way to create an open atmosphere is to model openness to the groups or individuals we are working with. Work through each activity yourself or with a trusted friend, before using it with your group, being willing to be vulnerable.

In any given moment we have two options: to step forward into growth or to step back into safety

Maslow
www.blobtree.com

The more we know ourselves the more others can know us too.

The activities are suitable for individuals, small groups or large ones. We've used Blobs with groups of thousands. Start small and build up your confidence to use them effectively. Never push people to reveal more than they want to. We all need to trust the groups we are in. This can take minutes or years, depending upon how well everyone gets on. Forcing people to step out beyond their comfort boundaries can lead to the opportunity for openness to close down right at the start. It is better to model it and allow others to take a similar risk.

Sharing our inner selves is a risk… but one worth taking.

General Questions to Ask Yourself and Others about the Blob Human Rights Resources

Which Blob:

1: …would you like to sit with?

2: …do you feel least like?

3: …do you feel like at the start of the week?

4: …is how you feel when you walk into your home?

5: …is how you felt at school?

6: …is how you felt yesterday?

7: …is how you feel about going on holiday?

8: …is how you feel when you wake up in the morning?

9: …is how you feel about God?

10: …is how you felt when you were bullied?

11: …is most like your mother?

12: …do you feel like at the end of the week?

13: …confuses you?

14: …is how you feel with children?

15: …is how you feel when you go to bed at night?

16: …is how you feel at a place of worship?

17: …is how you felt at the age of 5?

18: …is how you feel with adults?

19: …is how you feel when you are confronted by violence?

20: …is how you feel with animals?

21: …is when you last felt stupid?

22: …is most like your father?

23: …is how you felt at the age of 11?

24: …is how you feel about being photographed?

25: …is how you felt when you were last kissed?

26: …is how you feel going shopping?

27: …is how you feel when someone tells you off?

28: …do you feel like in a quiet place?

29: …is when you have to sort out an argument?

30: …is how you think you will feel at the age of 21?

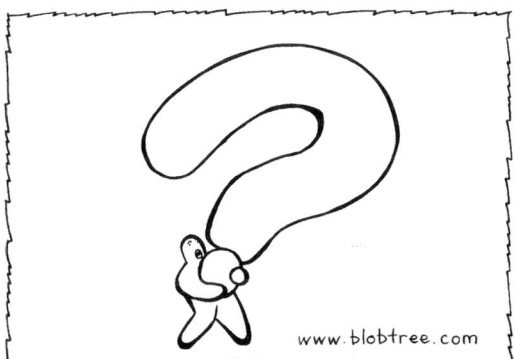

www.blobtree.com

31: …is when you get angry?

32: …is when you win a competition?

33: …is your brother or sister?

34: …is when you tell a lie?

35: …is when you go to a party?

36: …is how you feel when your parents are with you?

37: …is when someone points out your mistakes?

38: …is when you have free time?

39: …is how you feel about dying?

40: …is how you feel about going to hospital?

41: …reminds you of Christmas?

42: …is how you feel under pressure?

43: …is how you feel when you are under pressure to change

44: …is how you feel in a new group of people?

45: …is how you feel about getting older?

46: …is how you feel being with people who break the law?

47: …do you feel like when people ask you to help them?

48: …do you feel like today?

49: …reminds you of your best friend?

50: …is how you feel when in a car?

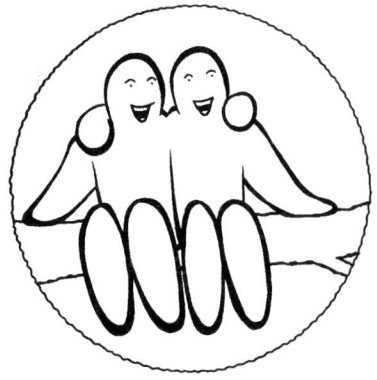

www.blobtree.com

Questions and the Blob Pictures

Questions are a very powerful tool. Those who work with people in education, law, care and personal development receive training in how to use them. A question such as, 'What can I do to solve the problem of poverty?' prompted Bob Geldof to initiate *Live Aid* and Bono to urge the G8 leaders to end international debt. Talking about our own thoughts and feelings enables us to understand where we are and where we need to change.

Can You Think of a Question Which Changed the Direction of Your Life?

Making time to talk about things in our heart has become part of the primary National Curriculum in 'circle time'. Counsellors are skilled in the art of both asking probing questions and listening to the spoken and unspoken responses so that they can ask further questions. Job interviews depend on questions and those who are skilled in how to answer them move on in their personal ambitions.

Church ministers use them to provoke us to think about our personal beliefs. Lawyers are trained in asking pertinent questions which expose the motives behind our actions and reveal what we don't want others to know about us. We all appreciate people who want to listen to our problems and ask us the questions that give us the space to talk.

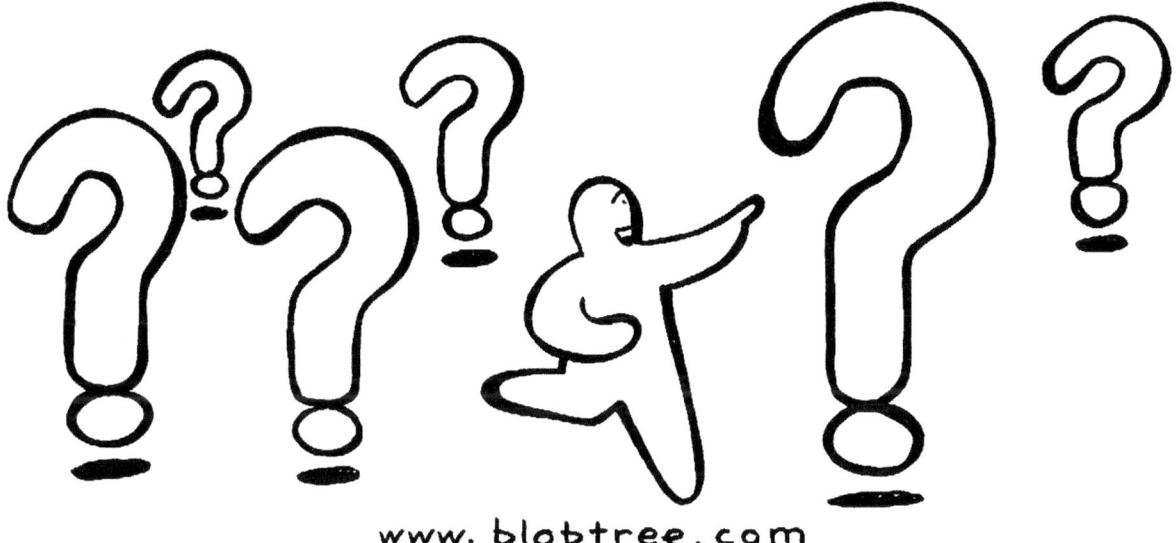

www. blobtree .com

Who Asks You the Best Questions in Your Life?

The most famous people in history were skilled at asking questions: Freud used them to reveal the thoughts of his clients; Jesus used them to expose the motives of religious hypocrites; Newton used them to understand the design of the universe; Mother Teresa used them to stir up the feelings of those who came to see her work with the world's poorest people; Martin Luther King, Jr. used them to challenge racist attitudes.

Are There Aspects of Your Work Which Would Be Improved by Asking More Questions?

There are different types of questions ranging from superficial ones (How you doing?) to deep and probing ones (What started you crying?). When you use the Blob pictures, remember that we all like to be questioned in a sensitive way. Sometimes we want to talk, and other times we like to listen. Start with general questions, and then enquire about your group's opinions, before finally giving them the opportunity to reveal the thoughts in their hearts. This whole process can happen the first time you meet together or it can take years.

When Did a Question Give You the Space to Come to Your Own Conclusion?

Valuing group members' response to the picture is essential. It enables the others to discuss more freely. There are no right or wrong answers. The Blobs provide your group with a chance to talk about an issue, or about themselves, using an image rather than a set of words. For some people it may be as simple as pointing at a picture to describe themselves; for others it will start a conversation full of stories.

Blob Questions – A Menu Approach

Add your own – these are just to start you off.

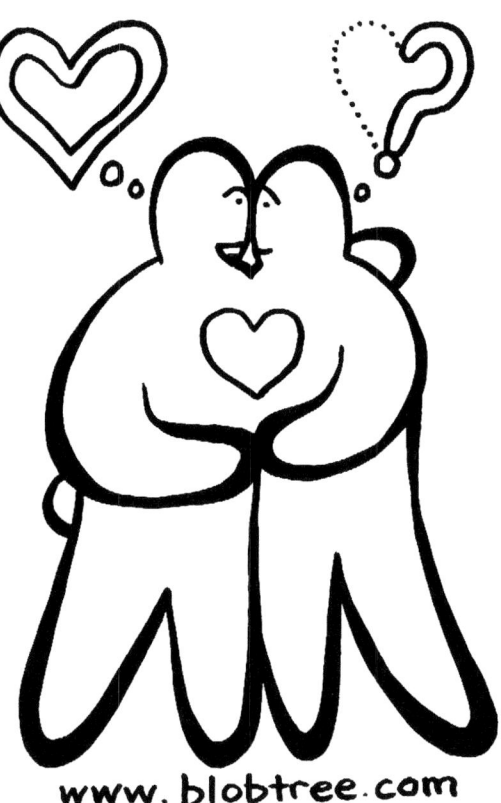

The menu approach for questions works well because it gradually builds trust and confidence between you and the person you are talking with. The first set of questions are general observations – factual. The second set are focused upon personal opinions. Don't get into conflicts here. If there are disagreements, simply remind them that the point of the Blobs is to share our opinions, and that there is no right or wrong answer. When the person you are working with is ready, move on to the third group – personal feelings. This process might take a matter of minutes or several sessions.

Starters (exploring general facts): Discuss with your partner what kind of feelings you can see. Which Blobs are on their own? Which Blobs are in groups? Which Blobs look happy? Which Blobs look sad? Find a Blob that interests you.

Main Course (exploring opinions): Which Blob is the most positive in your opinion? Which Blob is the most negative? Which Blob is like your teacher? Which Blob cares the most in your opinion? Which Blob do you not understand? Which Blob could be the leader? Which Blob is likely to be in trouble with the police? Which Blob could be working for the police? Which Blob could be rich? Which Blob is most likely to be taking drugs? Which Blob could die soon? Which is an old Blob? Which Blob is lonely?

Dessert (exploring feelings): Which Blob do you feel like? Which Blob would you like to be? Which Blob do you feel like when you've been drinking? Which Blob could God be? Which Blob could God not be? Which Blob scares you? Why? Which Blob reminds you of your mum? Which Blob reminds you of your dad? Which Blob is the friend you've always wanted? Which Blob would you keep away from? Which Blob annoys you the most? Why?

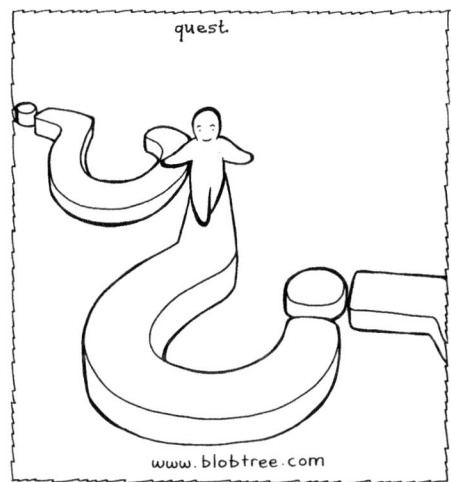

Blob
Trees

CHILDREN'S HUMAN RIGHTS

Introduction to Blob Trees

When we originally designed the Blob Tree, in the early 1980s, it was as something that could be used with all people, focusing upon feelings. At that time, Pip was working with young people who struggled to express themselves, and so he conceived the idea of a visual solution – an image that could be pointed at to overcome the limitations of language or confidence.

Late one evening, we created the first drawing on a thin piece of card, with spiky branches, clumsily drawn Blobs, searching for appropriate feelings to be depicted. Initially the Blobs had noses, but then we realised that these were unnecessary to convey body language and so liquid paper edited them out. We were trying to find the simplest way to illustrate feelings and behaviour. Pip trialled this with young people at The Mayflower, a family centre in the East End of London where he worked, and found that it was effective as a tool.

The Blobs were drawn without age, gender, clothes or any limiting features. They could be used globally as the two languages they utilise are feelings and body language, common to us all, the world over. The Tree represents a group, such as a family, a workplace, a class or organisation. It was the simplest natural structure that we could imagine to house our Blobs.

As you use these different trees to reflect upon human rights issues, remember that this is not just an exercise in facts and opinions. For many of the people you are working with, these issues impact upon their friends and family. Feelings are so important to encourage if we are to recognise the way that abuses of human rights make us all suffer. If the human rights matter to us, then they need to matter to children and adults across the world.

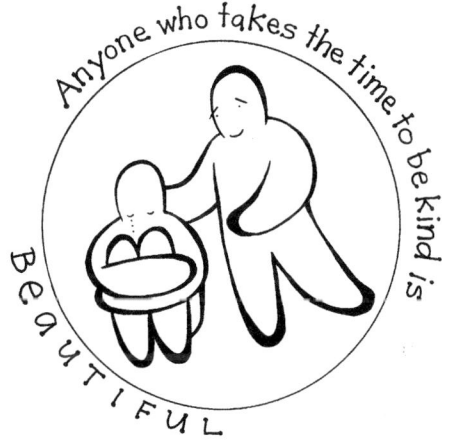

Anyone who takes the time to be kind is Beautiful

www.blobtree.com

Some of these images contain behaviour which is both violent and cruel. This is not to celebrate it, but to enable the children to talk about how they might have been physically and emotionally attacked. It is important to help children and adults to discuss painful topics in a safe and appropriate way. Please use your professional judgement as to when it would be suitable to introduce the different visual tools, and regarding the suitable group size.

Human Rights Blob Tree

Look at the Human Rights Blob Tree.

What kinds of behaviour can you see?

Which human rights articles can you identify? (the list from pp. 48–9 may help here)

What feelings can you identify?

Which Blobs look like helpers?

Which Blobs have you felt like?

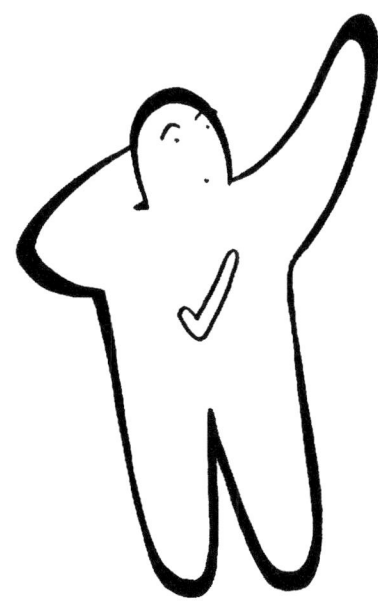

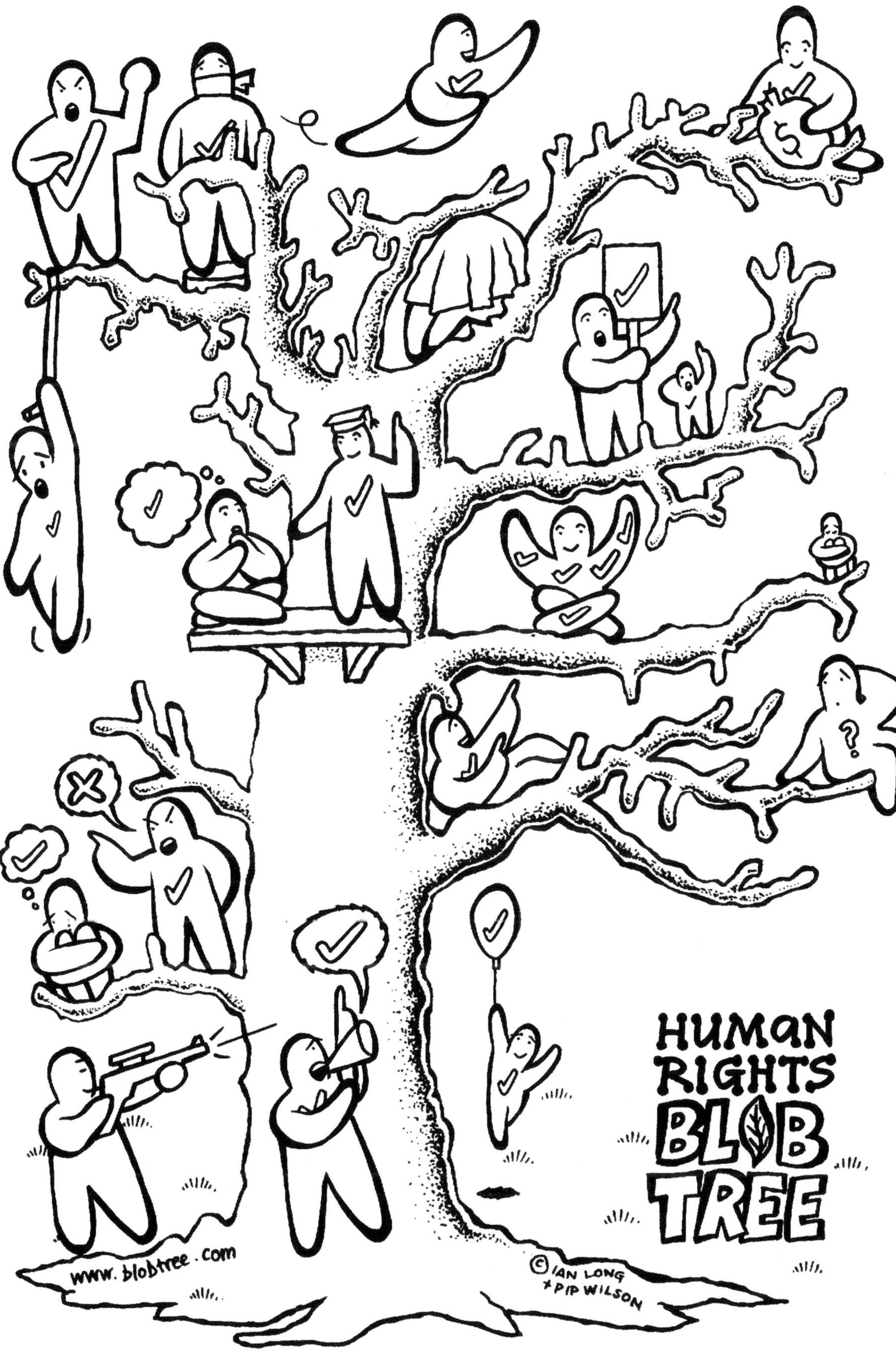

Responsibility Blob Tree

Look at the Responsibility Blob Tree.

What kinds of behaviour can you see?

What feelings can you identify?

Which Blobs are being responsible?

Which Blobs have you felt like?

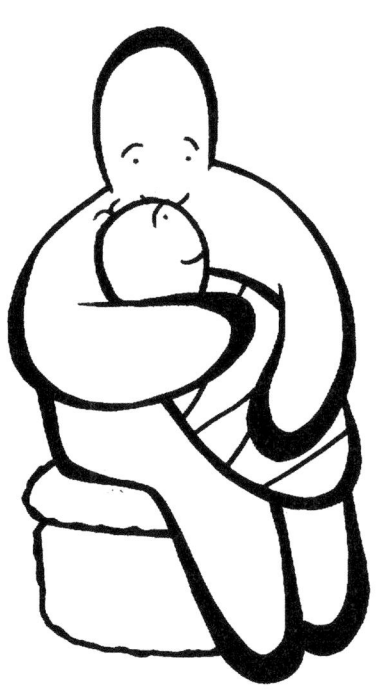

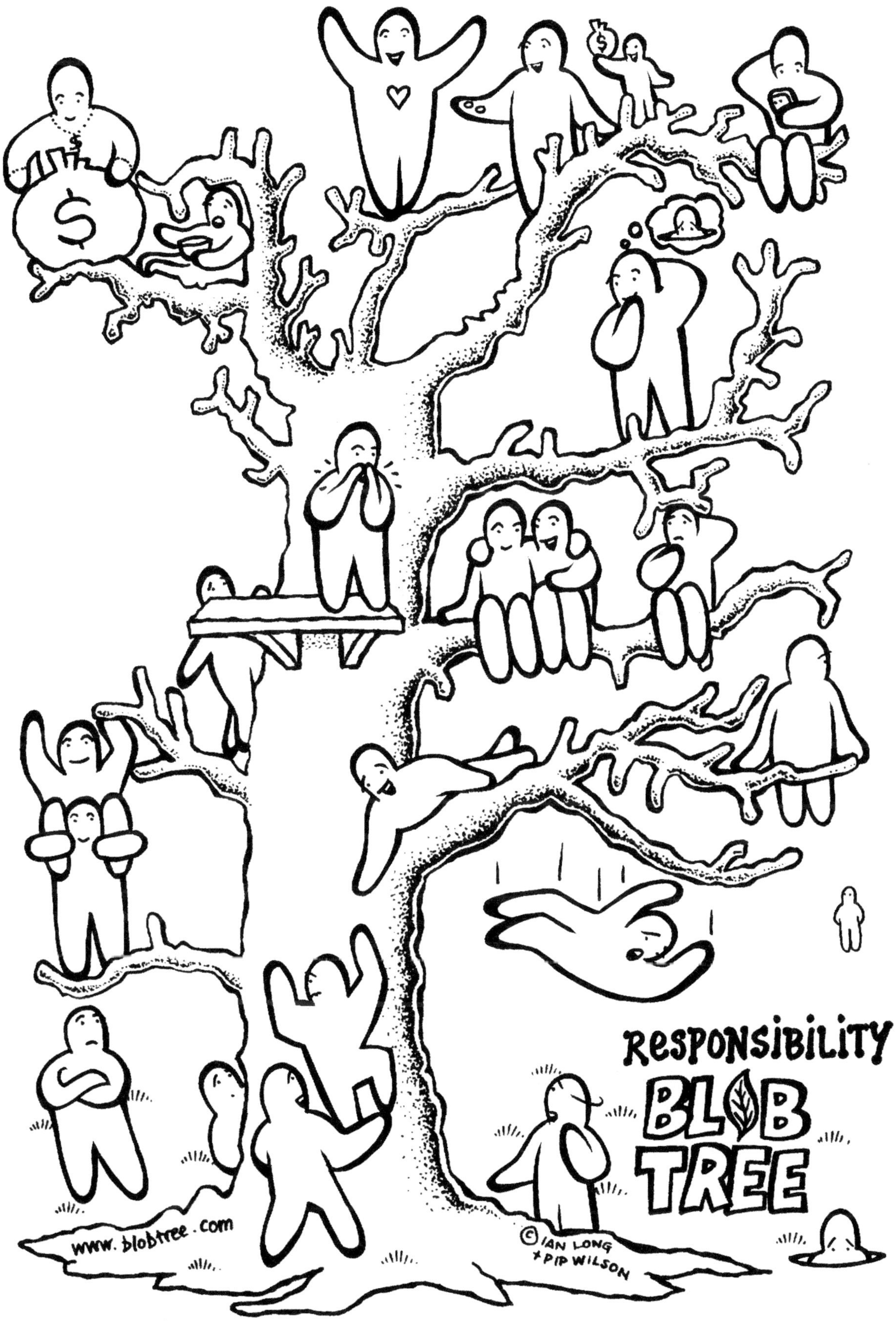

www.blobtree.com

RESPONSIBILITY
BL🍃B
TREE

©IAN LONG
+PIP WILSON

Disability Blob Tree

Look at the Disability Blob Tree.

What kinds of disability can you see?

What feelings can you identify?

Which Blobs need immediate help?

Which Blobs have you felt like?

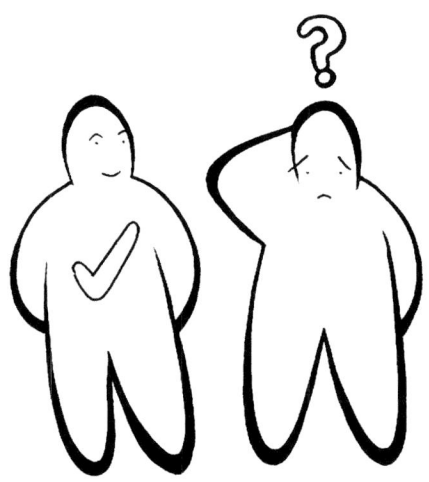

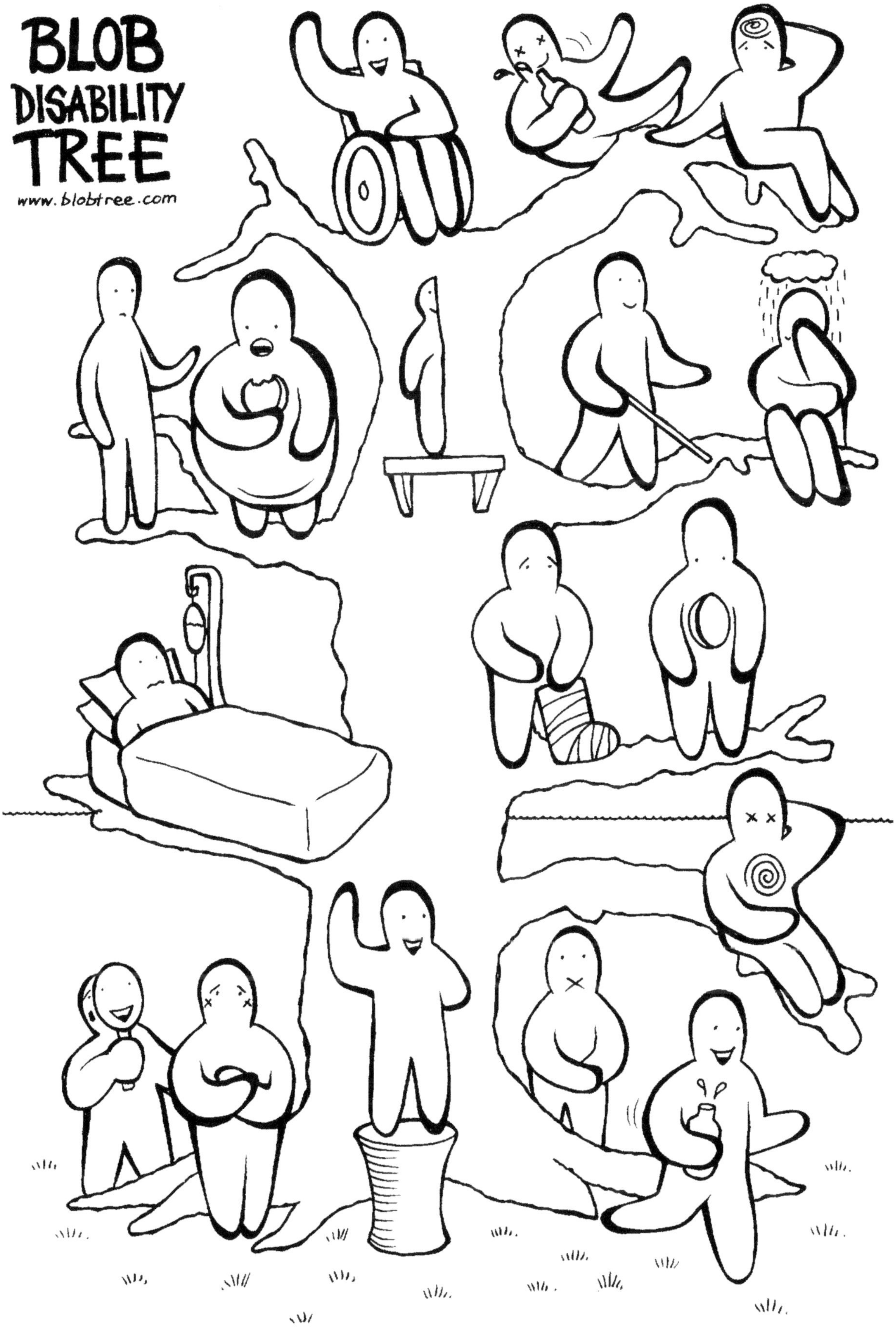

BLOB
DISABILITY
TREE
www.blobtree.com

COMPANION @ WEBSITE

Free Speech Blob Tree

Look at the Free Speech Blob Tree.

What kinds of behaviour can you see?

What feelings can you identify?

Which Blobs are able to speak their mind freely?

Which Blobs have you felt like?

Which Blobs would most benefit from support?

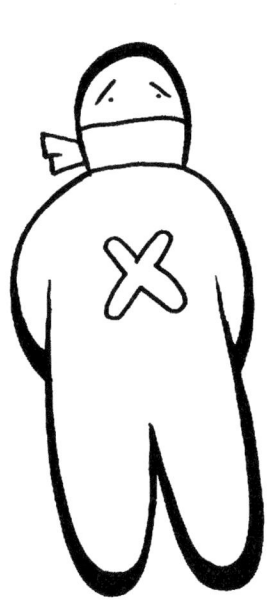

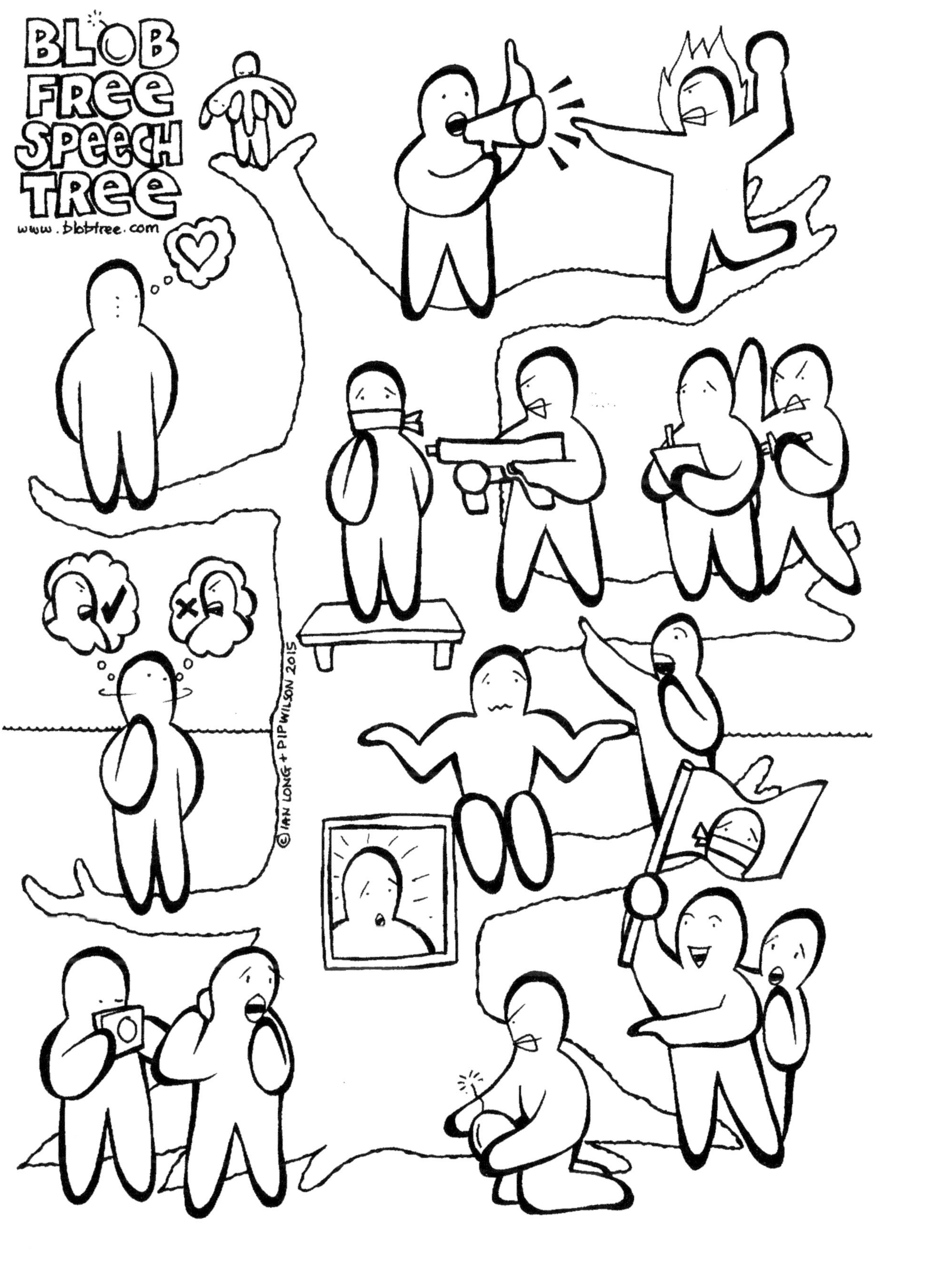

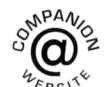

CHILDREN'S HUMAN RIGHTS

Privilege Blob Tree

Look at the Privilege Blob Tree with your talk partner.

What kinds of behaviour can you see?

What feelings can you identify?

Which Blobs are the privileged?

Which Blobs have you felt like?

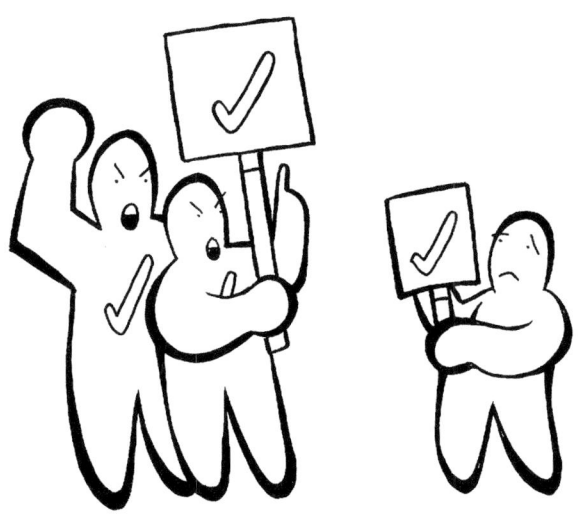

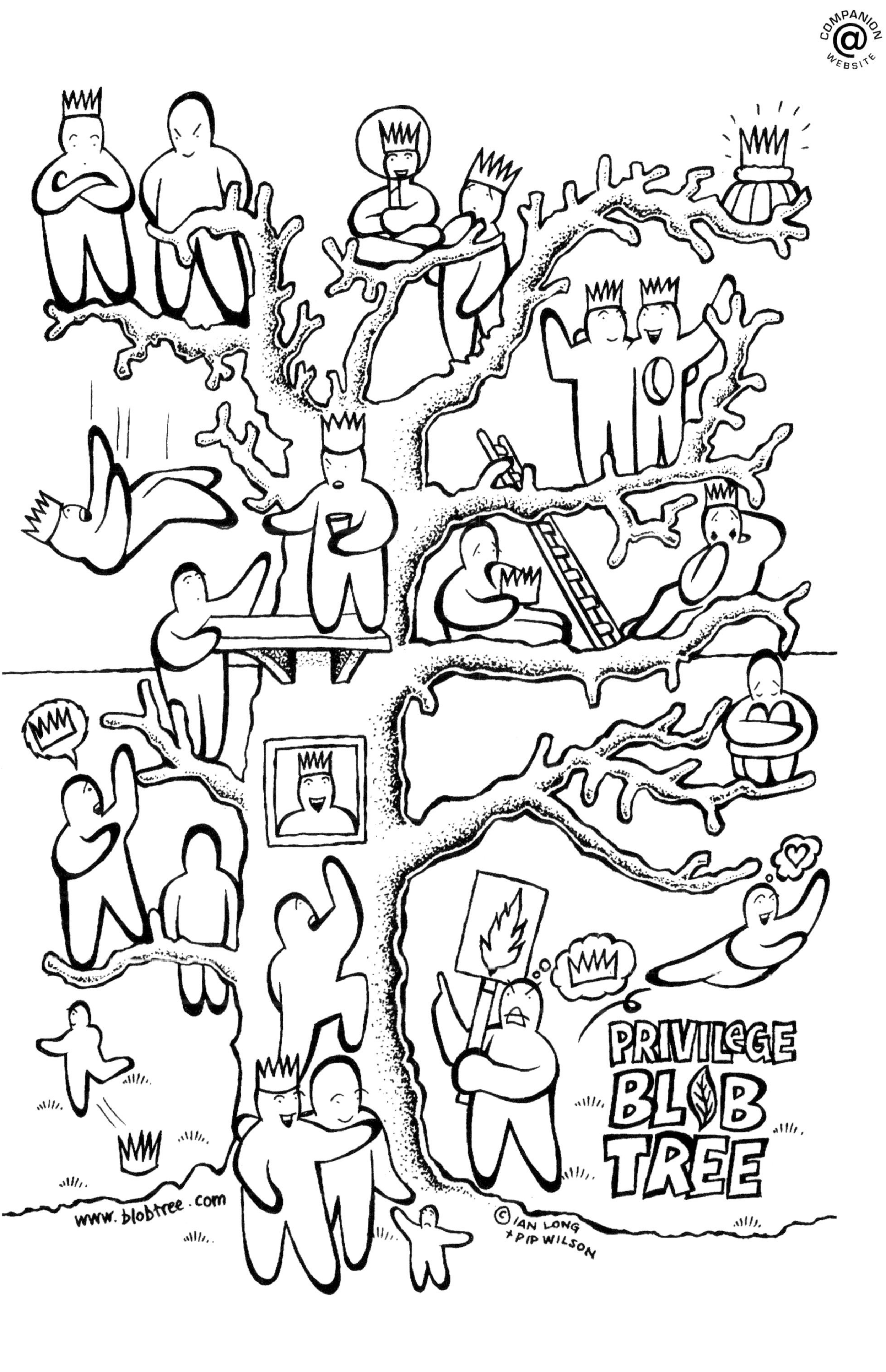

Kindness Blob Tree

Look at the Kindness Blob Tree.

What acts of kindness can you see?

What feelings can you identify?

Which Blobs have you felt like?

Which Blob is most in need of kindness?

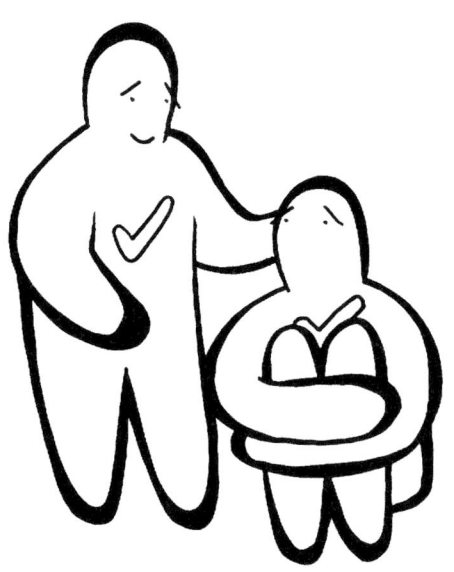

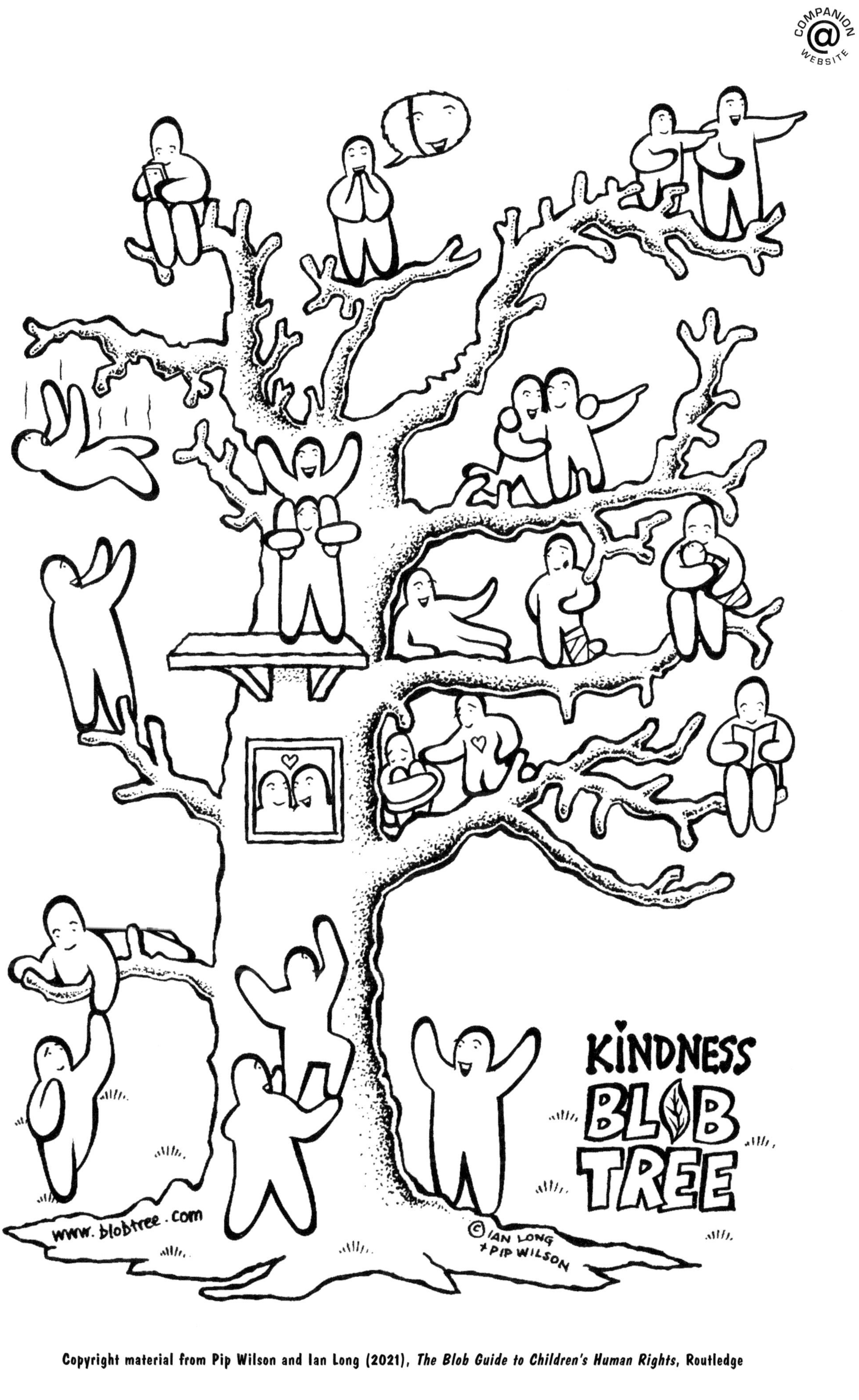

Copyright material from Pip Wilson and Ian Long (2021), *The Blob Guide to Children's Human Rights*, Routledge

Unkind Blob Tree

Look at the Unkind Blob Tree.

What kinds of behaviour can you see?

What could these images symbolise (see below)?

What feelings can you identify?

Which Blobs are being very unkind?

Which Blobs have you felt like?

Which human rights articles can you identify that are being broken (see pp. 48–9)?

Some aspects of this image may upset younger children. It would not be suitable for children who do not understand symbolism, for example. Talking through what the children perceive would be helpful. No one has big scissors that cut a person in half, for example, but some people use their words to hurt and scare others.

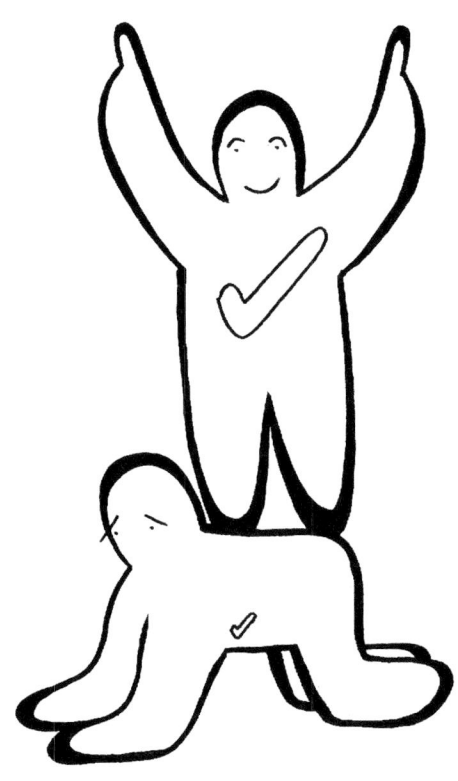

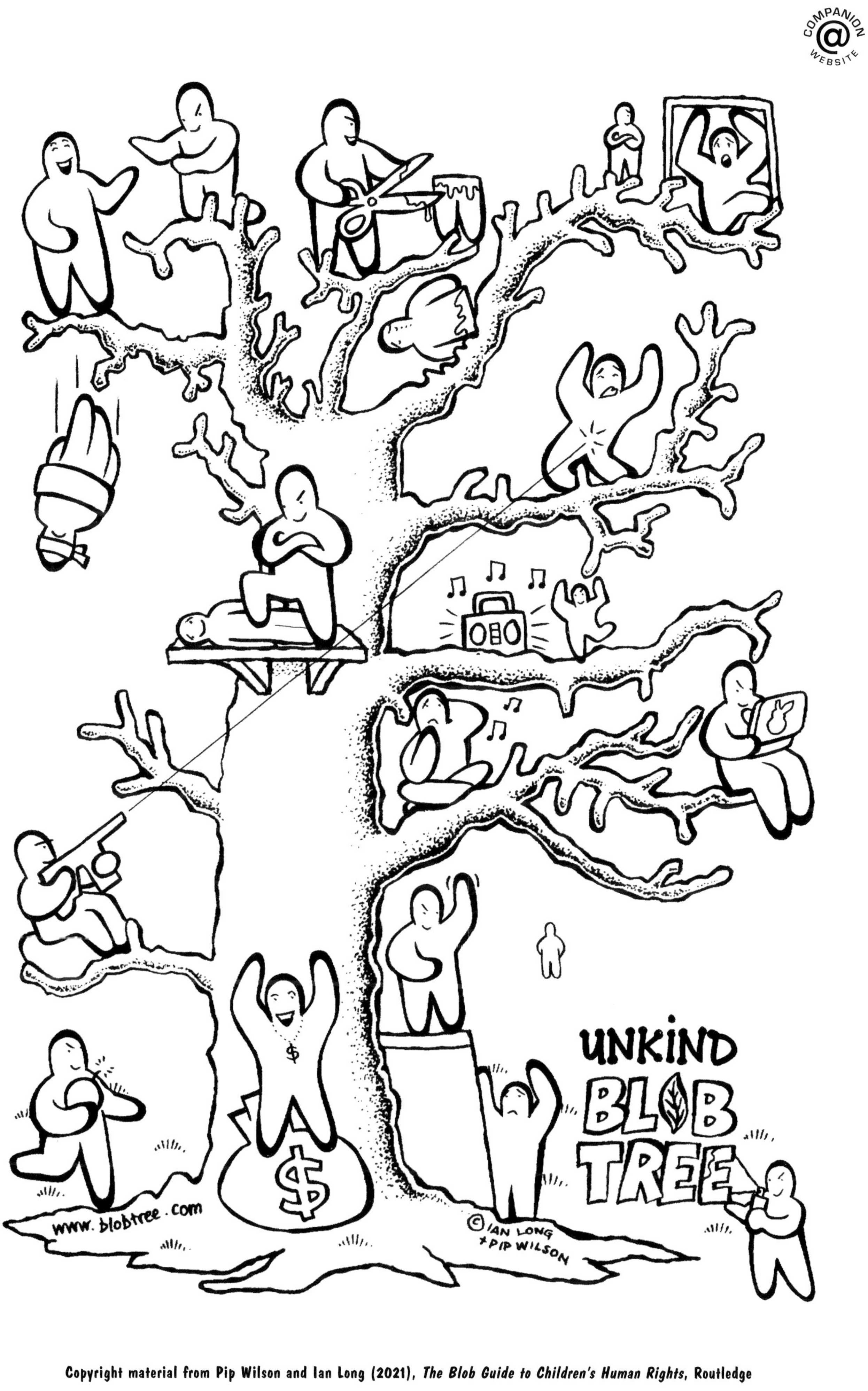

UNKIND
BLOB
TREE

www.blobtree.com

© IAN LONG + PIP WILSON

Listening Blob Tree

Look at the Listening Blob Tree.

What kinds of behaviour can you see?

What feelings can you identify?

Which Blobs are listening well?

Which Blobs have you felt like recently?

Which Blobs would you like to be more like?

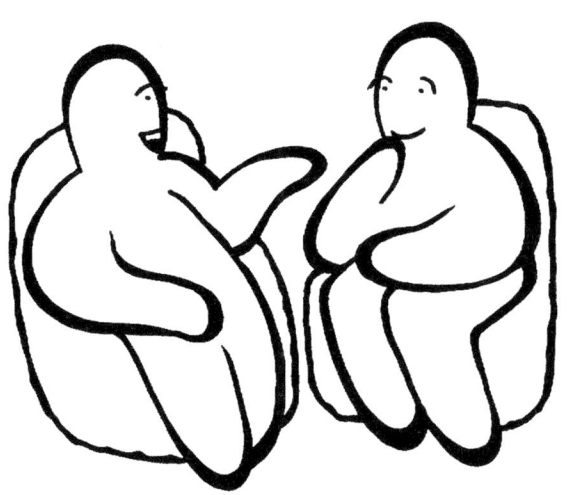

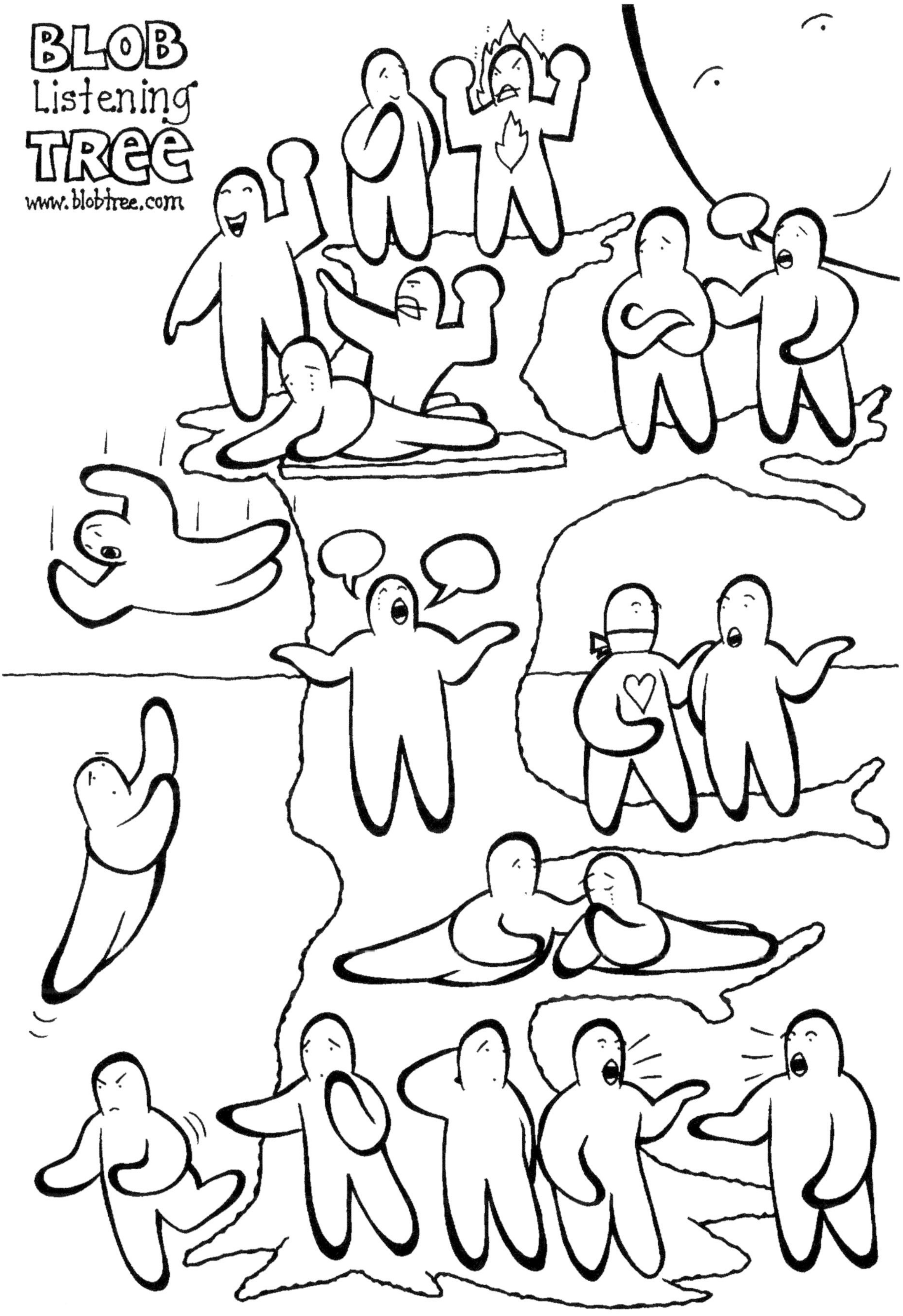

BLOB
Listening
TREE
www.blobtree.com

Drawing the Line.

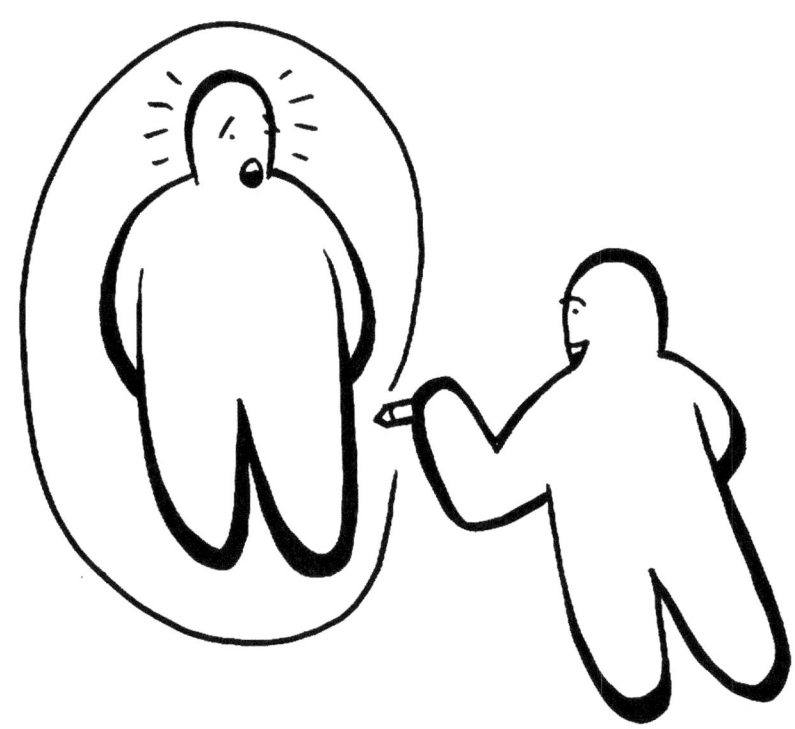

Drawing the Line

The following set of Blob tools are scales from high to low (or vice versa). They enable questions to be asked alongside the images. Here is an example of how to use them with the 'Listening' tool. Below are three instructions which can either be verbally asked, which is the best way, so that the Blobs are the main focus, or written underneath the image if your group are fully literate. We wouldn't recommend giving written instructions to primary-aged pupils as so many struggle with the reading and comprehension elements of the question.

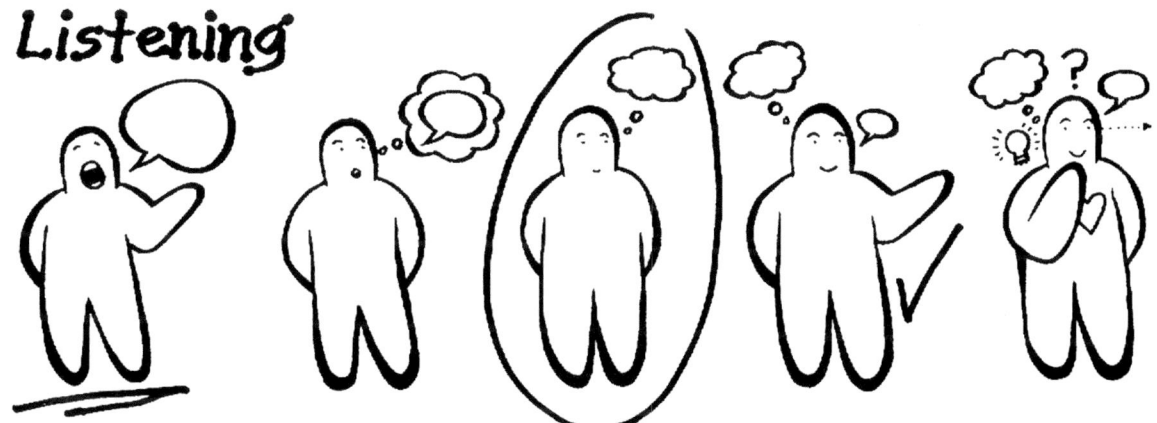

Circle the Blob that shows how well you listen to instructions
Tick the Blob that shows where you would like to aim to be
Underline the Blob that shows how well you listen in group work

Ian: Here's how I would use this image in a classroom or with a group, for example. I would project the image up on an interactive screen, and provide the children with their own paper copy/digital image. Make sure that they add their name! Explain that today we are looking at a skill that some will be very good at already, and others can identify where they need to improve. Emphasise that it's okay to not be good at everything.

Discuss with them the two end Blobs – the talker and the careful listener. Give them examples of what both extremes might represent in the context that you are assessing. Also discuss the middle Blob and how that one is somewhere between the two. I would model how I would answer the first question, including my thinking aloud, so they can see the process I'm going through, as well as the line I draw.

Ask if anyone has a question before they circle their first answer. Remind them to be as honest as they can be so that it helps them to assess themselves accurately. Display the question on the board after asking it again.

Then repeat the process for the second and third questions. If the group work well together, get them to share with a partner where they assessed themselves to be and to explain why. This is to help with their justification, not so that their partner can correct what marks they've made.

Invariably, the first few goes may be wildly inaccurate. What you might see is not how good at listening they are, or whatever subject you've chosen, but rather how they feel about themselves. Those who are more self-aware might gravitate to a humbler Blob, whilst those with lots of self-confidence might be well above their pay grade! Over time, this will change, as they begin to see that accurate self-assessments enable them to see where they are currently, and the next step to take.

For each theme, we have added three exemplar questions, but please write your own that are appropriate for your age, context and theme being explored.

CHILDREN'S HUMAN RIGHTS

Drawing the Line – Human Rights

Circle the Blob that shows how well you know the forty-two human rights

Underline the Blob that shows how much you talk about human rights

Tick the Blob that shows how important human rights are to you in your own country

Drawing the Line – Responsibility

Circle the Blob that shows how much you tidy and clean at home

Underline the Blob that shows how much you clear away after a meal and do the washing up

Tick the Blob that shows how responsible you are at school

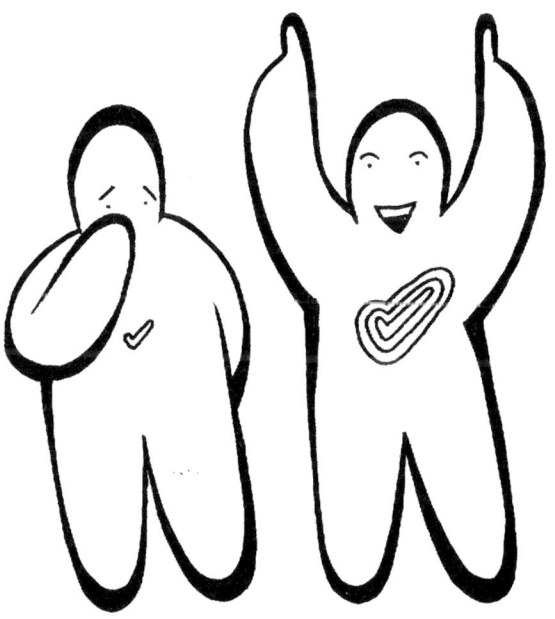

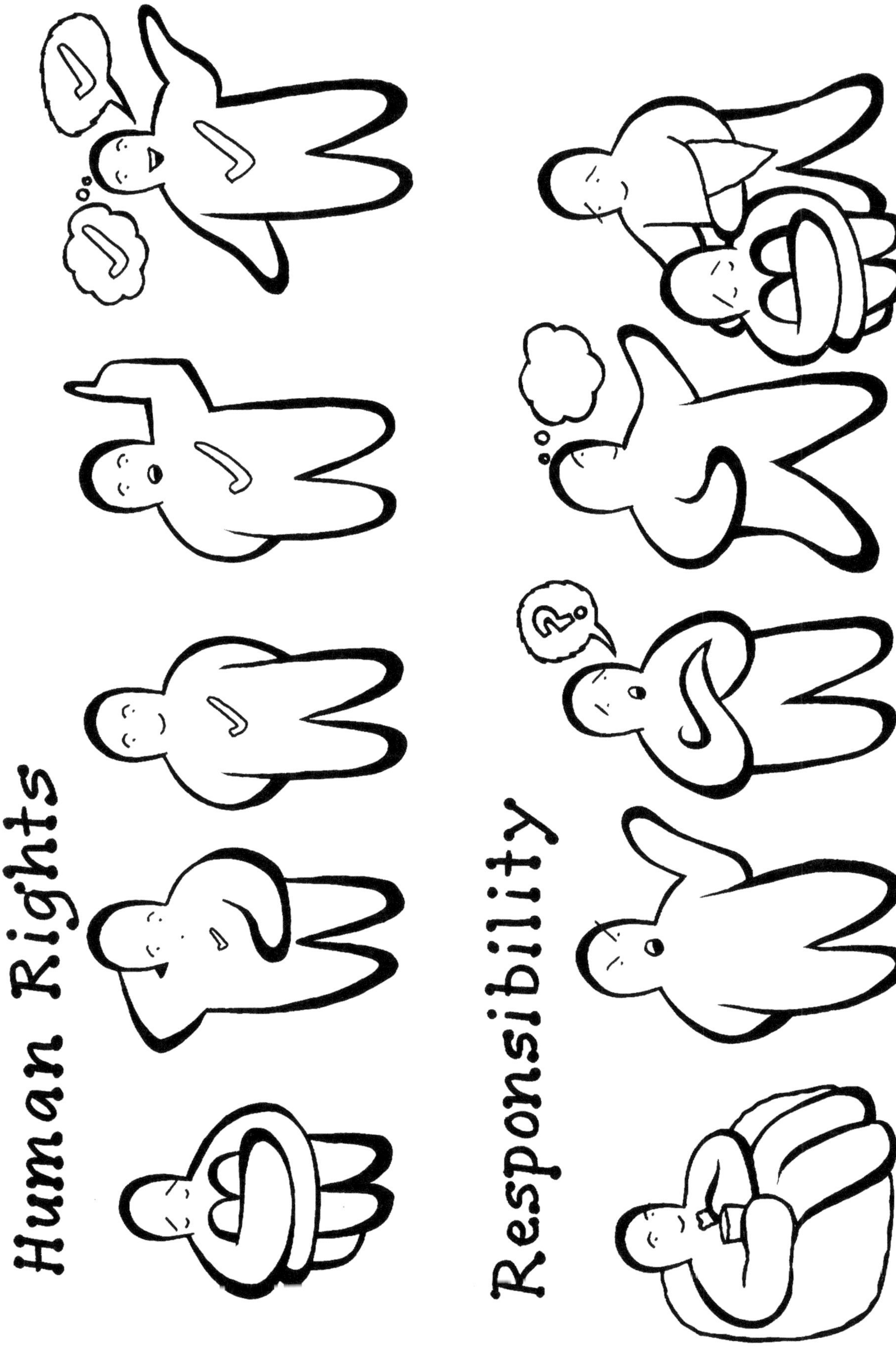

Human Rights

Responsibility

Drawing the Line – Giving

Circle the Blob that shows how much you enjoy giving gifts to friends

Underline the Blob that shows how much you give gifts to strangers

Tick the Blob that shows how important giving people your time is

Drawing the Line – Touching

Circle the Blob that shows the type of touch you experience most at school

Underline the Blob that shows the type of touch you experience most at home

Tick the Blob that shows the type of touch that you like the most

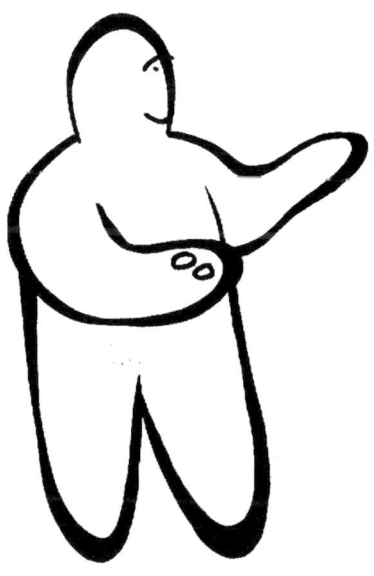

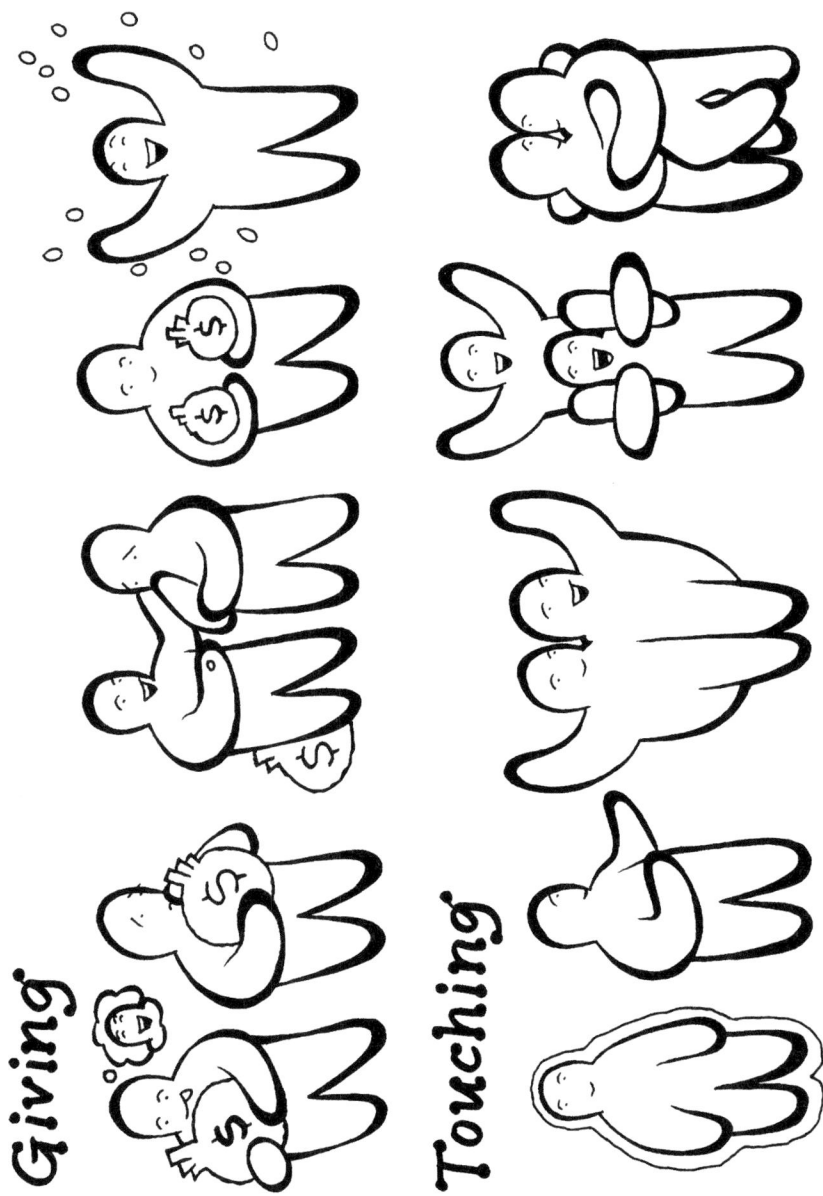

CHILDREN'S HUMAN RIGHTS

Drawing the Line – Freedom of Religion

Circle the Blob that shows how free you feel to practise your beliefs at school

Tick the Blob that shows the level of freedom you want for your beliefs

Underline the Blob that shows the level of freedom you would allow everyone if you were in charge of your country

Drawing the Line – Protection

Circle the Blob that shows how well protected you feel at home

Underline the Blob that shows how well protected you feel at school

Tick the Blob that you have never felt like

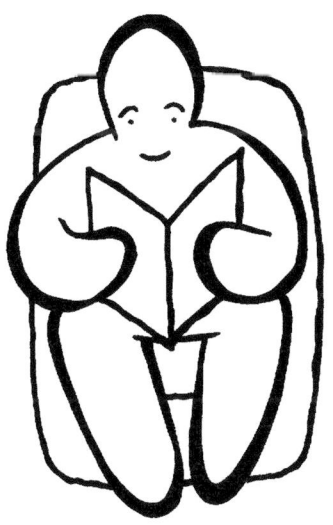

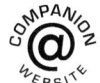

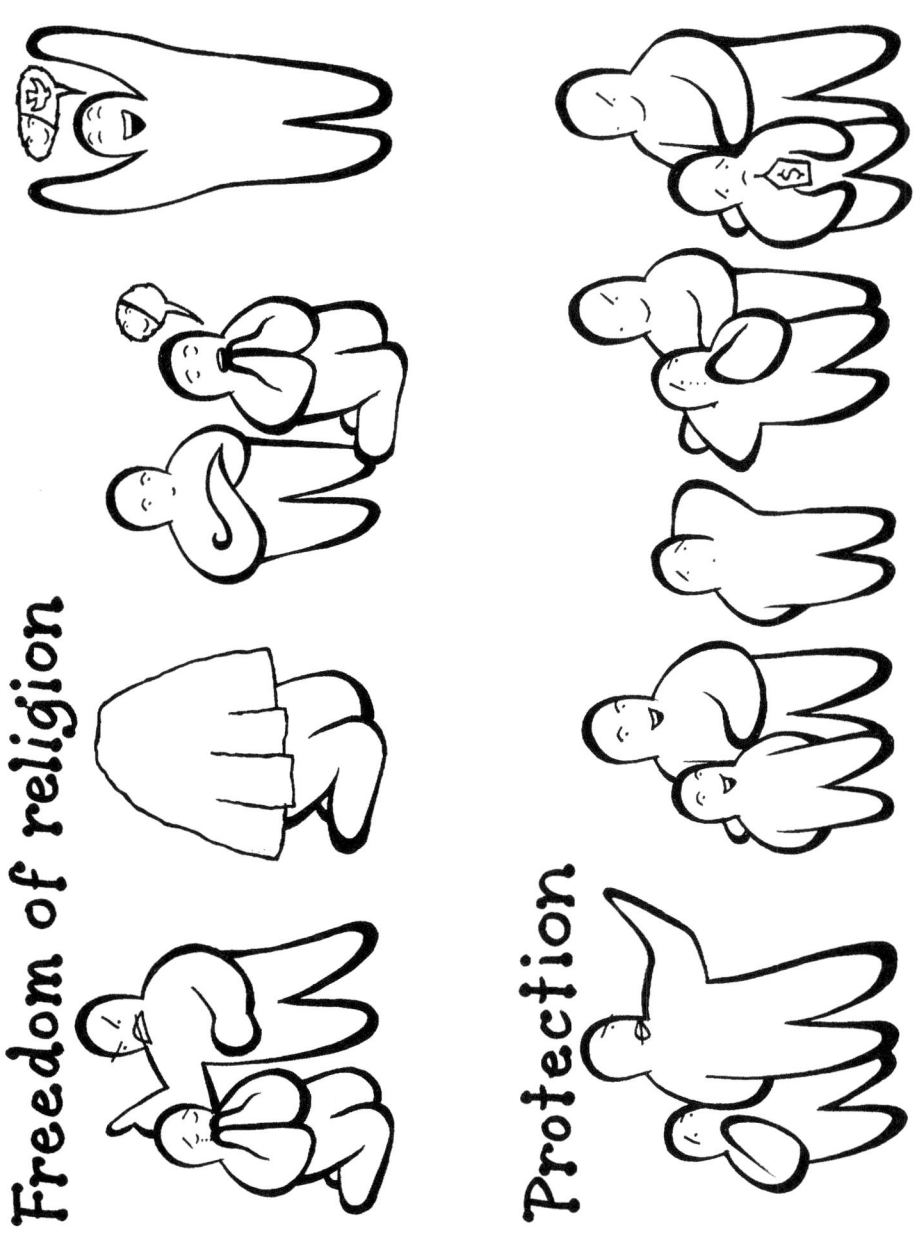

Freedom of religion

Protection

CHILDREN'S HUMAN RIGHTS

Drawing the Line – Inclusion

Circle the Blob that shows how included you feel in the playground

Underline the Blob that shows how included you feel at home

Tick the Blob that shows how included you feel when you are lonely

Drawing the Line – Having a Voice

Circle the Blob that shows how confident you are to answer questions in class

Underline the Blob that shows how confident you are to say how you feel

Tick the Blob that shows how confident you are to speak out against bullies

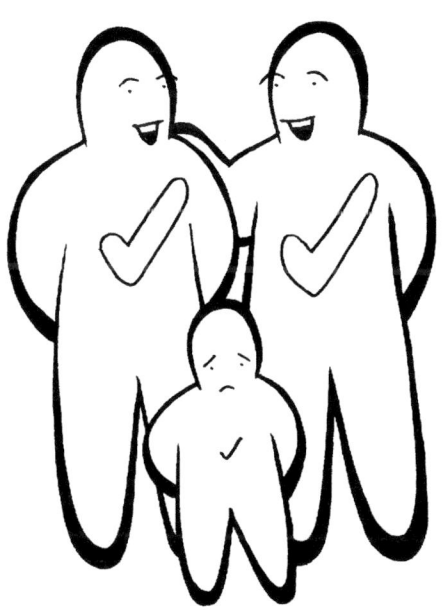

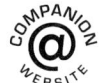

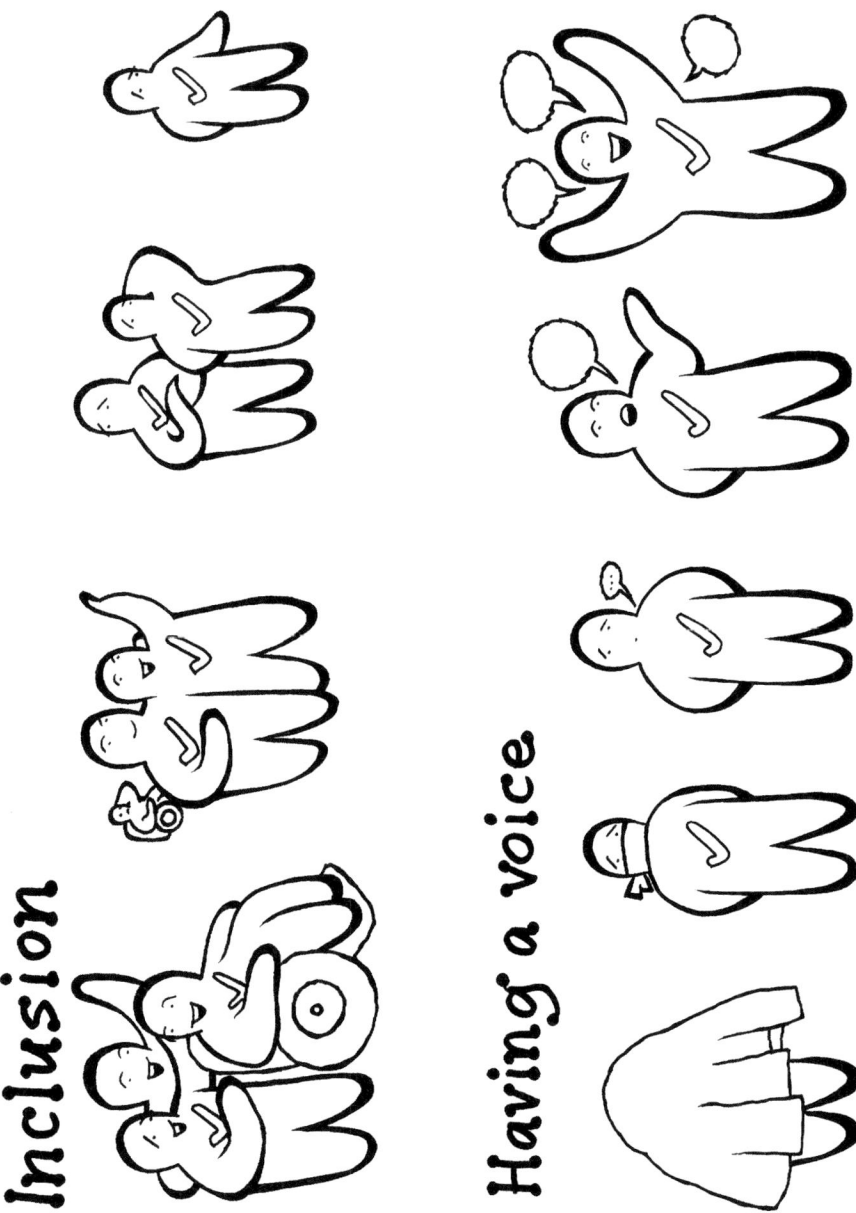

Inclusion

Having a voice

CHILDREN'S HUMAN RIGHTS

Drawing the Line – Access to Information

Circle the Blob that shows how much you enjoy searching for information

Underline the Blob that shows your favourite approach to searching for information

Tick the Blob that shows how easy it is to get information at school

Drawing the Line – Right to Play

Circle the Blob that shows how easy it is to play with others at school

Underline the Blob that shows how easy it is to play at home

Tick the Blob that shows how easy it is to play on holiday

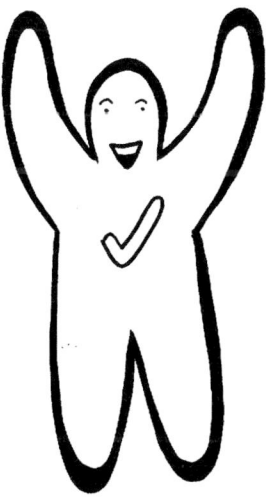

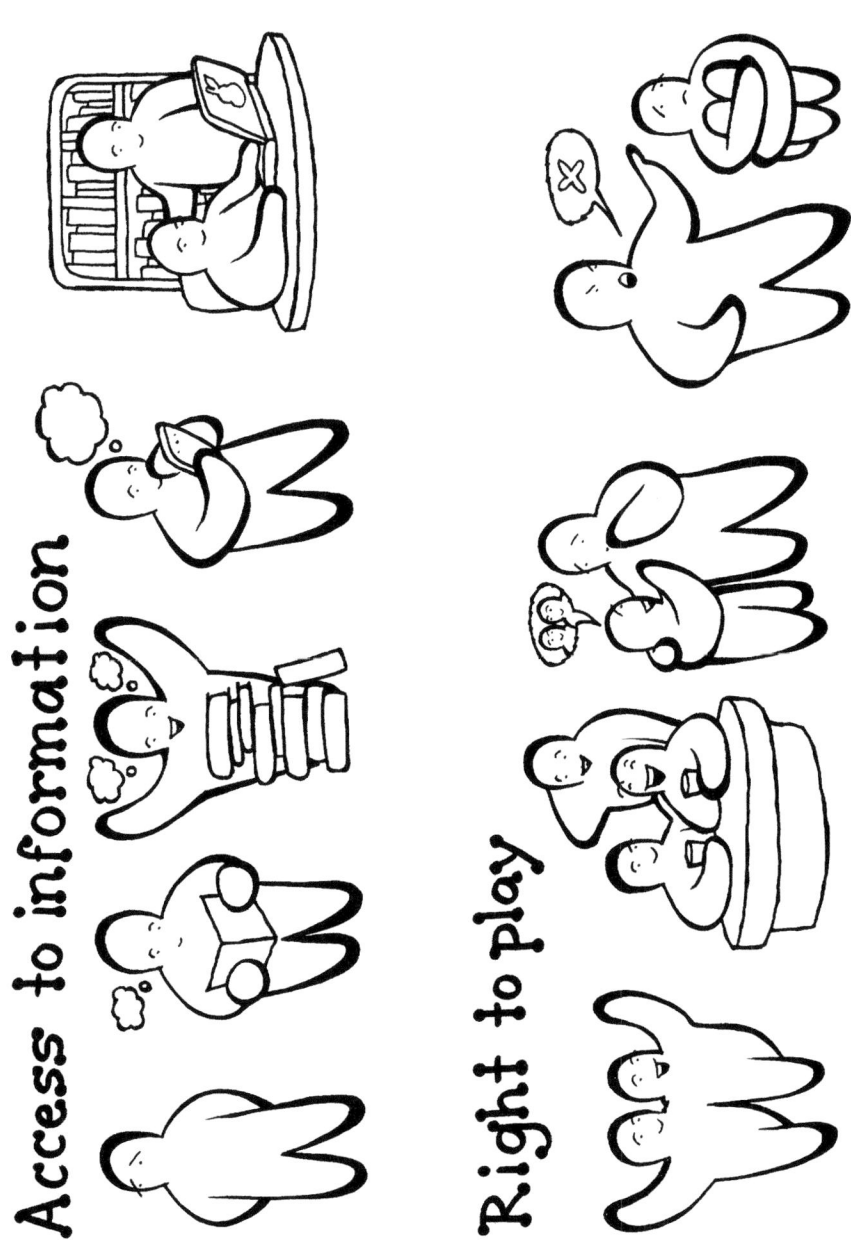

Access to information

Right to play

CHILDREN'S HUMAN RIGHTS

Drawing the Line – Helpful

Circle the Blob that shows how you like to be helped

Underline the Blob that shows how you help others at school

Tick the Blob that shows how you help your family at home

Drawing the Line – Generous

Circle the Blob that shows how you spend or share your pocket money or birthday money

Underline the Blob that shows how you would like your friends to share their money with you

Tick the Blob that shows how you would share your money with someone who had no money of their own

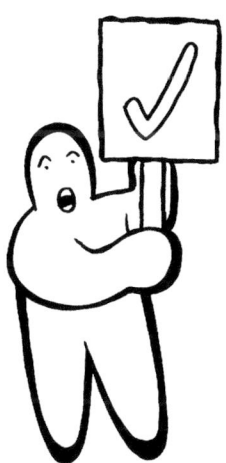

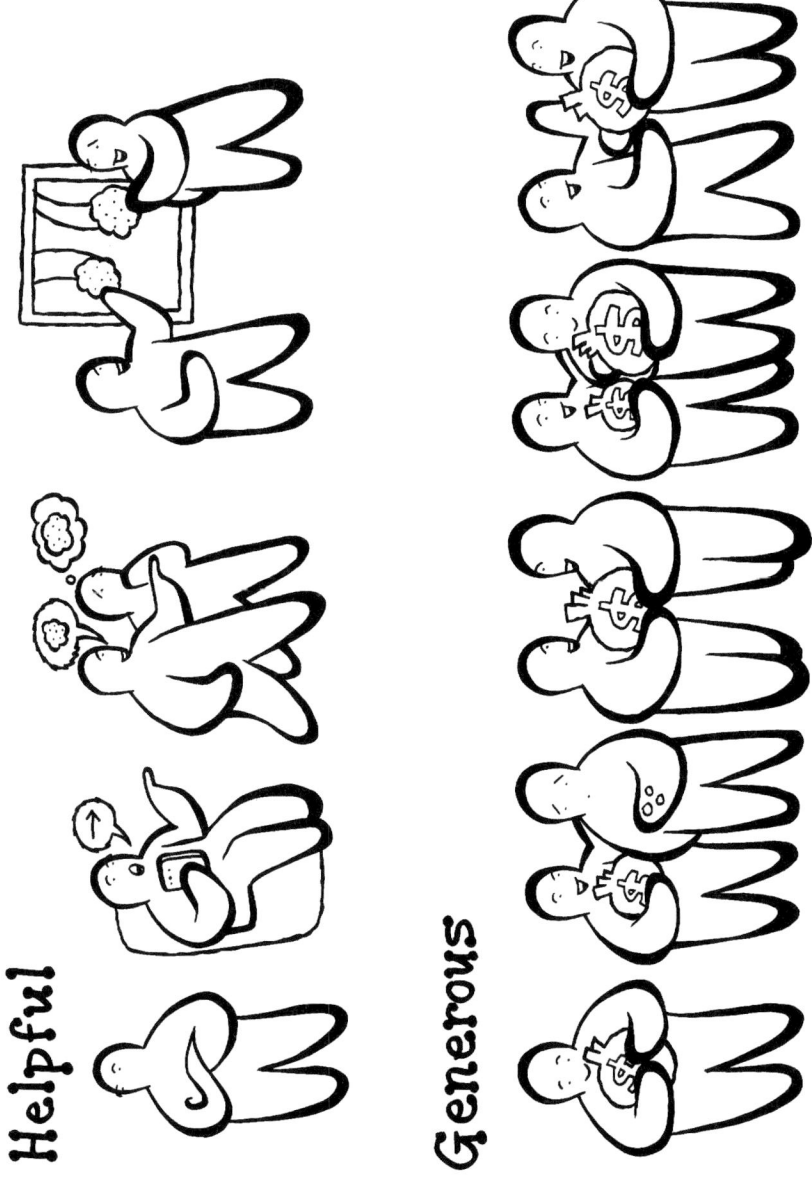

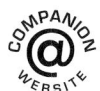
Drawing the Line – Freedom of Movement

Circle the Blob that shows how free you are to go and wander at school

Underline the Blob that shows how free you would like to be as a child

Tick the Blob that shows how free you would like to be as an adult

Drawing the Line – Right to Life

Circle the Blob that shows your current age

Underline the Blob that society values the least by its actions

Tick the Blob that shows the best age to be alive

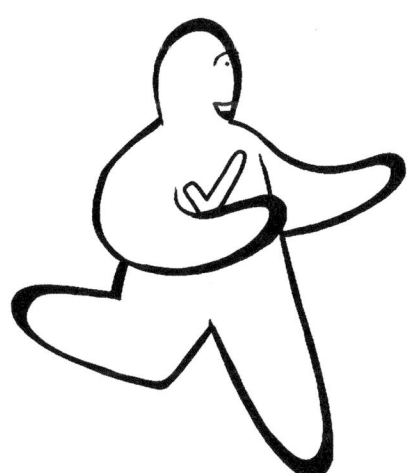

Freedom of movement

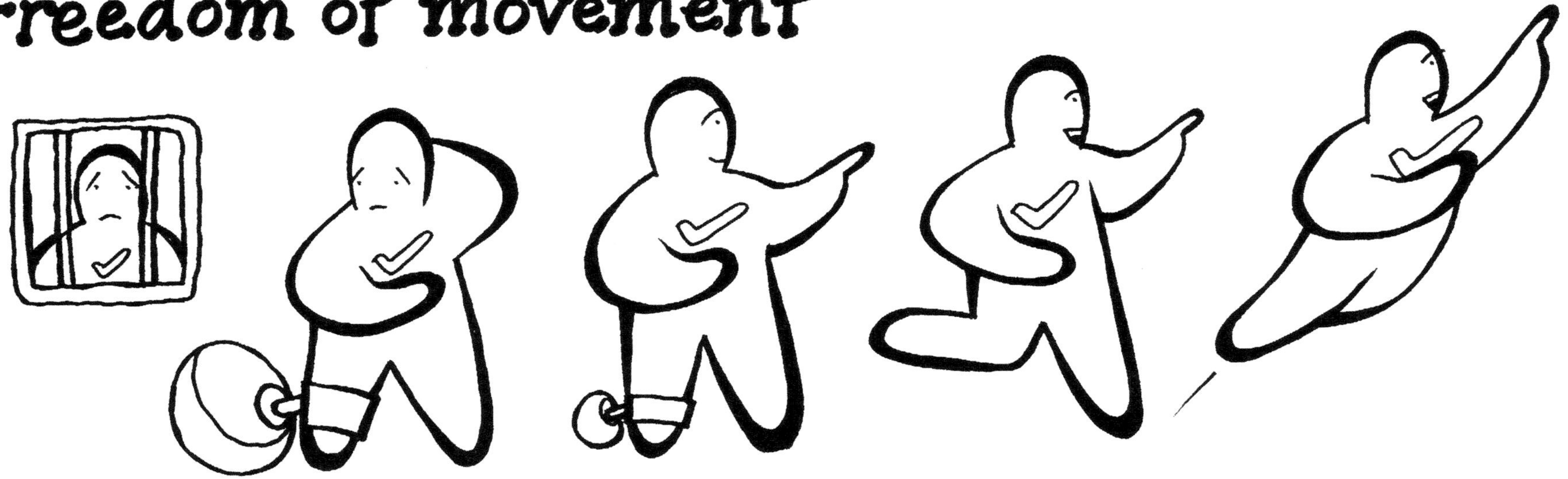

Right to life

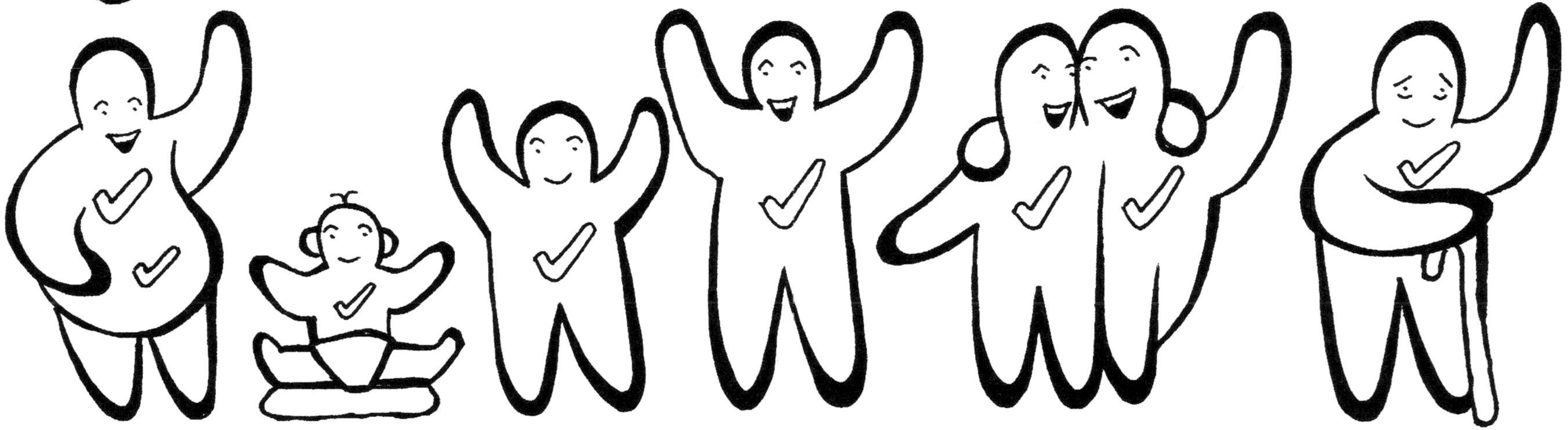

CHILDREN'S HUMAN RIGHTS

Drawing the Line – Safety

Circle the Blob that shows how safe you feel most of the time

Underline the Blob that shows how safe you feel at night

Tick the Blob that shows how safe you feel without an adult around

Drawing the Line – Appropriate Housing

Circle the housing that you would enjoy most in the summer

Underline the housing that you would dislike to be in during winter

Tick the housing that you have never experienced

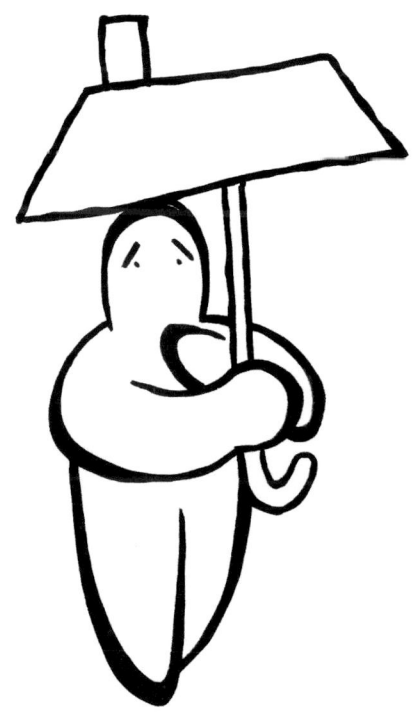

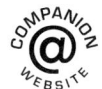

Safety

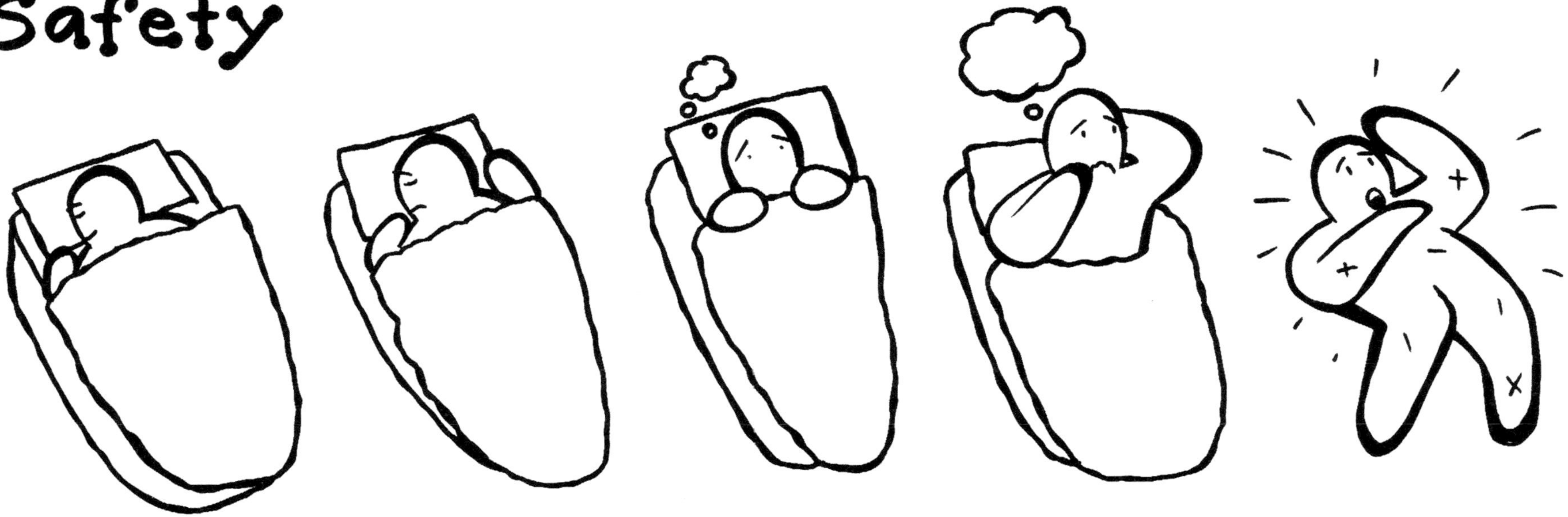

Appropriate housing

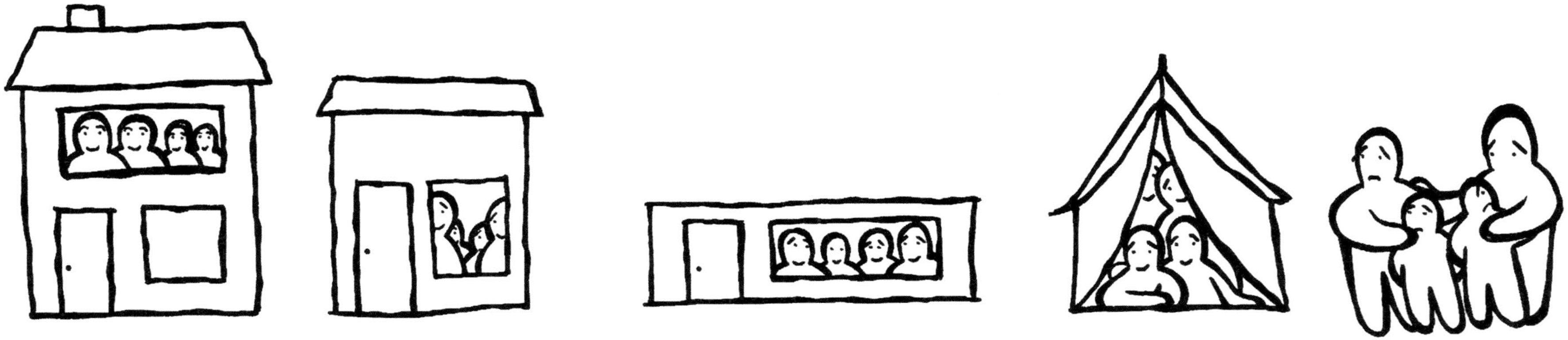

Drawing the Line – Education

Circle the Blob that shows the type of education you enjoy

Underline the Blob that shows how you have never felt about learning

Tick the Blob that shows the feeling most of your friends have about education

Drawing the Line – Appropriate Punishment

Circle the Blob that shows how you think children should be punished

Underline the Blob that shows how you think adults should be punished

Tick the Blob that shows the worst way you've been punished at school

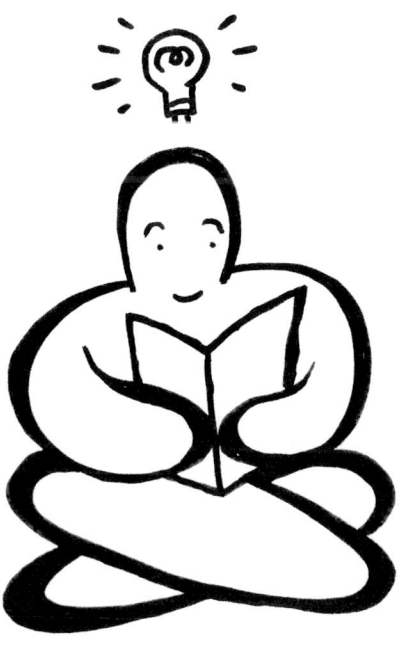

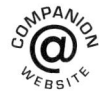

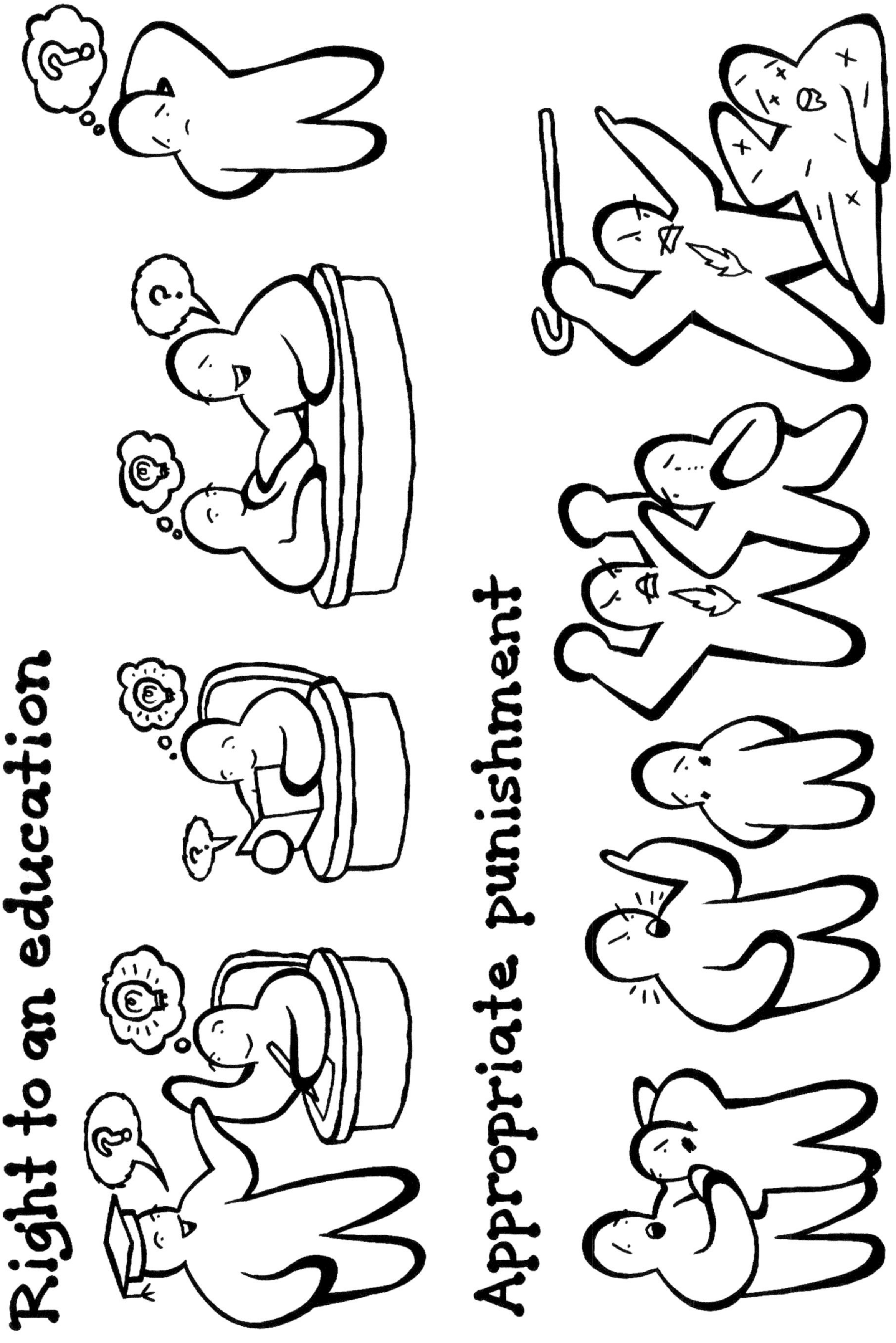

Right to an education

Appropriate punishment

Blob
Human
Rights
Articles

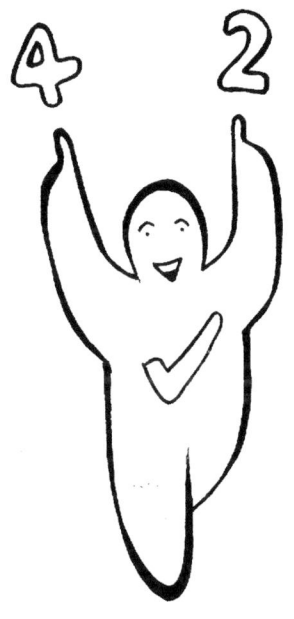

CHILDREN'S HUMAN RIGHTS

The Forty-Two Children's Rights Articles

When Ian was working with Heathfield School, one of the boys, Sazhad, had rewritten the forty-two articles in a simpler way. He took notice of these simpler explanations alongside the official definitions, and then created each of the images for the articles.

The Rights from the United Nations Convention on the Rights of the Child

Every child has the right to have rights [Article 1]

Every child has the right to equality [Article 2]

Every child has the right to have their best interests considered [Article 3]

Every child has the right to have their rights respected by governments [Article 4]

Every child has the right to have family guidance [Article 5]

Every child has the right to live and grow [Article 6]

Every child has the right to know and be cared for by their parents if possible [Article 7]

Every child has the right to know their identity [Article 8]

Every child has the right to be cared for safely by both parents even if they live apart [Article 9]

Every child has the right to keep in contact with both parents if they live abroad [Article 10]

Every child has the right to live in the country they are supposed to stay in [Article 11]

Every child has the right to be heard [Article 12]

Every child has the right to have a say [Article 12]

Every child has the right to express their opinions [Article 13]

Every child has the right to think about different religions [Article 14]

Every child has the right to practise a religion [Article 14]

Every child has the right to meet friends, unless there is a good reason not to [Article 15]

Every child has the right to private times [Article 16]

Every child has the right to trustworthy information [Article 17]

Every child has the right to family support from their government [Article 18]

Every child has the right to be safe [Article 19]

Every child has the right to be looked after with consideration for their culture [Article 20]

Every child has the right to have their best interests prioritised if they are adopted [Article 21]

Every child has the right to the same rights as other children if they become a refugee [Article 22]

Every child has the right to be treated with dignity if they have a disability [Article 23]

Every child has the right to take part [Article 23]

Every child has the right to a clean environment [Article 24]

Every child has the right to the best possible health [Article 24]

Every child has the right to have their well-being checked regularly if they're not living with family [Article 25]

Every child has the right to appropriate housing, food and clothing [Article 26]

Every child has the right to a reasonable standard of living [Article 27]

Every child has the right to learn [Article 28]

Every child has the right to an education [Article 28]

Every child has the right to be treated in ways respectful of their dignity [Article 28]

Every child has the right to be their best [Article 29]

Every child has the right to care for the world [Article 29]

Every child has the right to speak their own language [Article 30]

Every child has the right to follow their own family's way of life [Article 30]

Every child has the right to play and relax [Article 31]

Every child has the right to take part in a variety of activities [Article 31]

Every child has the right to be protected from harmful work [Article 32]

Every child has the right to be protected from bad drugs [Article 33]

Every child has the right to be protected from being touched in uncomfortable or upsetting ways [Article 34]

Every child has the right to be protected from being taken away illegally [Article 35]

Every child has the right to be protected from harmful activities [Article 36]

Every child has the right to be protected from inappropriate punishment [Article 37]

Every child has the right to be protected from taking part in wars if they are aged under 15 [Article 38]

Every child has the right to special help if they have been hurt or ignored [Article 39]

Every child has the right to be treated fairly if they do something wrong [Article 40]

Every child has the right to change if they do something wrong [Article 40]

Every child has the right to keep their rights in their country [Article 41]

Every child has the right to know that they have r ights [Article 42]

How to Use These Images

Each image can be photocopied onto its own piece of paper so that those reflecting upon its meaning can annotate it and apply it to school, family and national life.

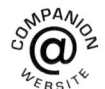

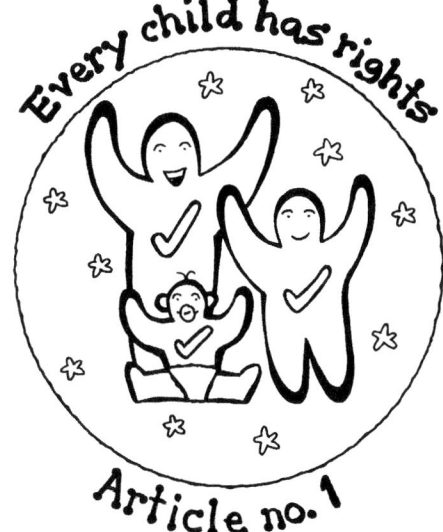

Every child has rights

Article no. 1

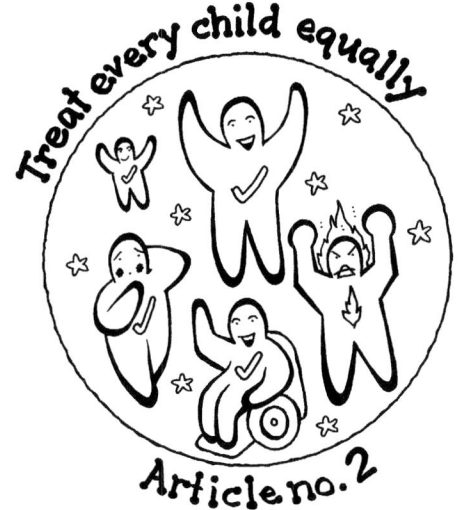

Treat every child equally

Article no. 2

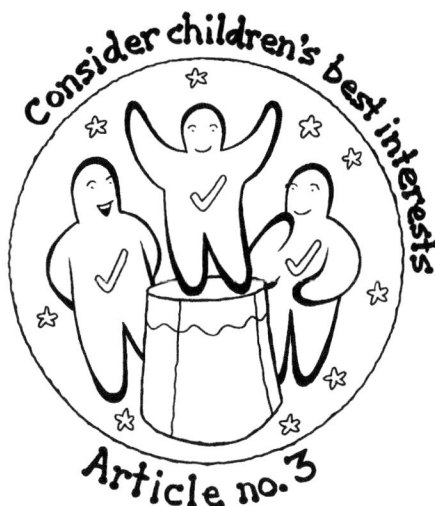

Consider children's best interests

Article no. 3

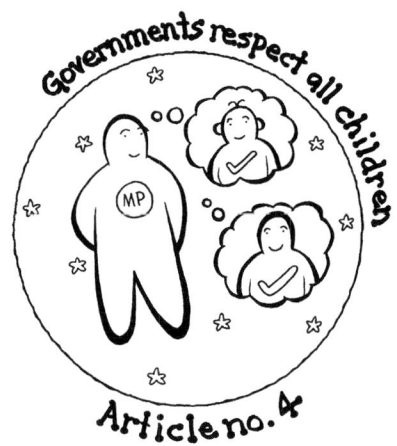

Governments respect all children

Article no. 4

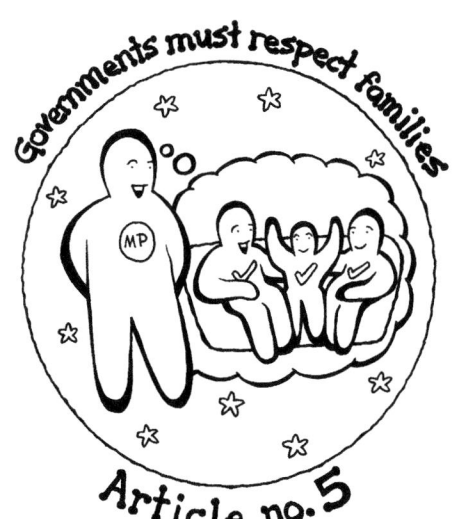

Governments must respect families

Article no. 5

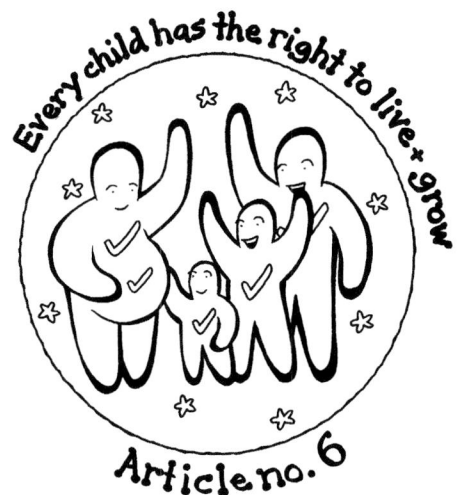

Every child has the right to live + grow

Article no. 6

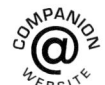

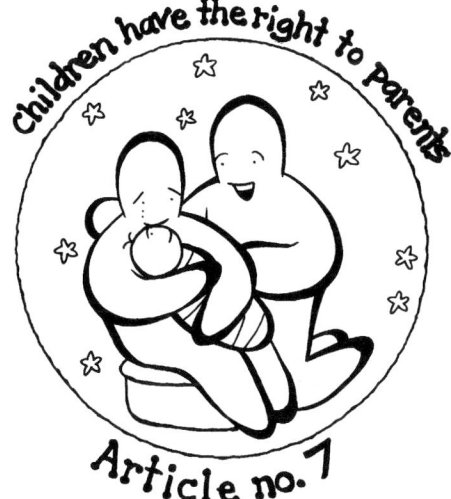

Children have the right to parents

Article no. 7

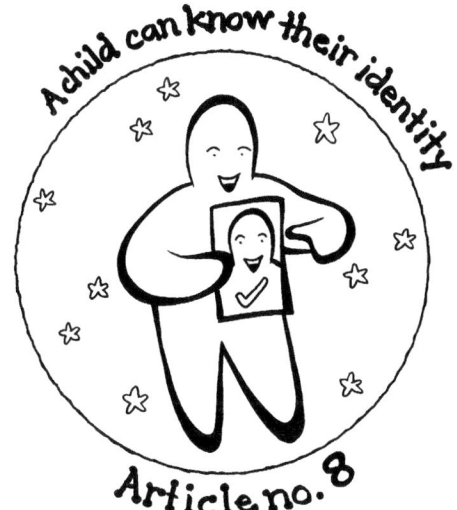

A child can know their identity

Article no. 8

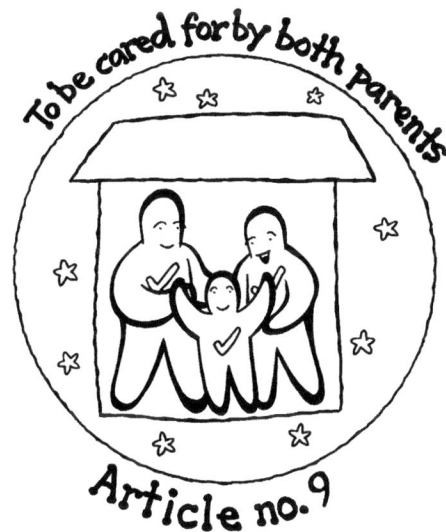

To be cared for by both parents

Article no. 9

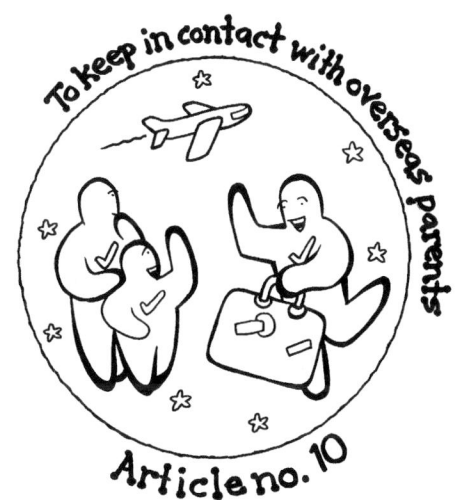

To keep in contact with overseas parents

Article no. 10

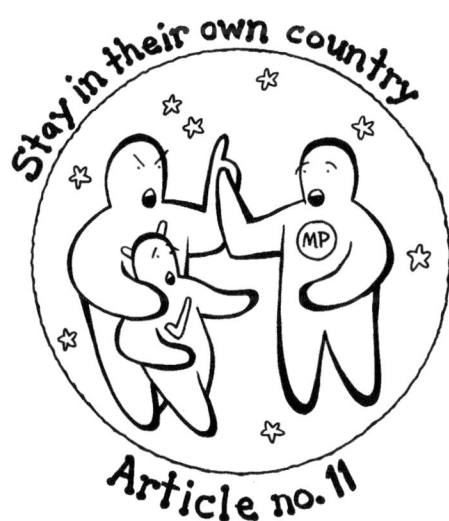

Stay in their own country

Article no. 11

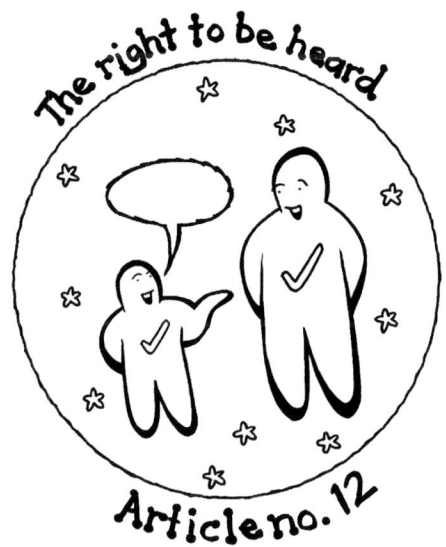

The right to be heard

Article no. 12

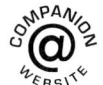

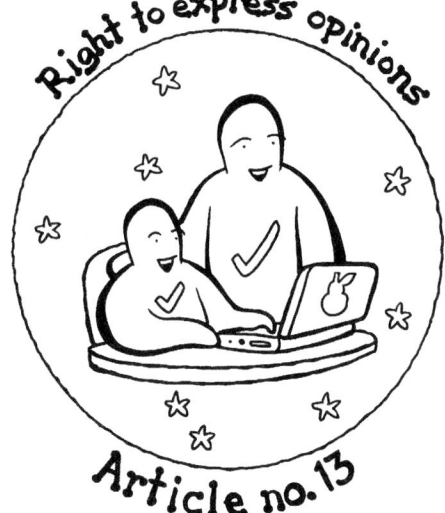

Right to express opinions

Article no.13

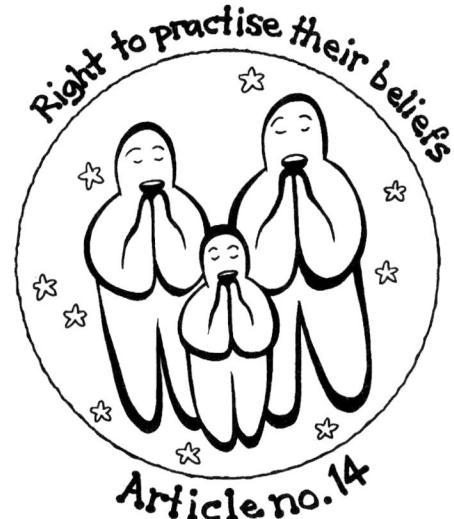

Right to practise their beliefs

Article no.14

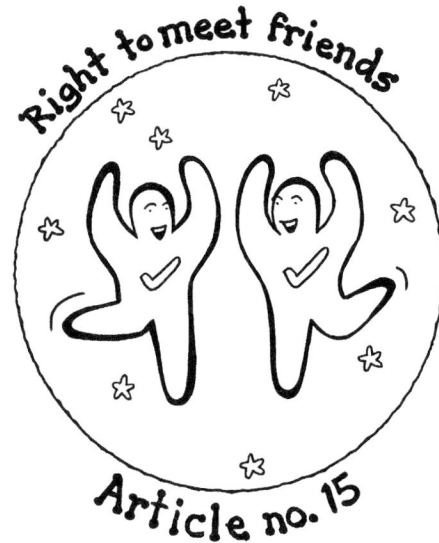

Right to meet friends

Article no.15

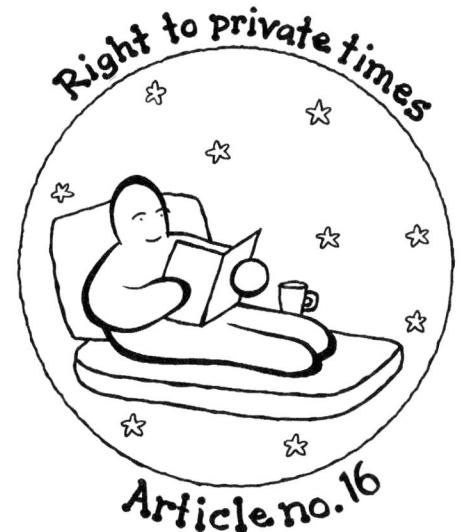

Right to private times

Article no.16

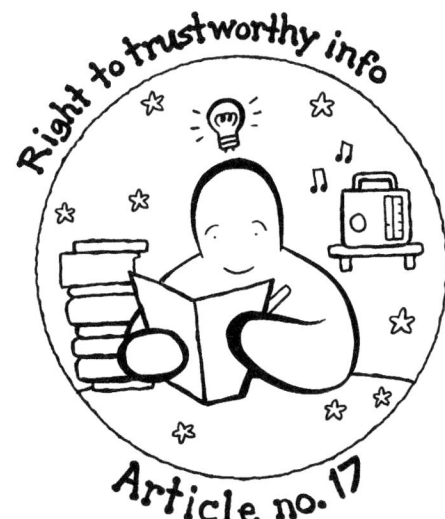

Right to trustworthy info

Article no.17

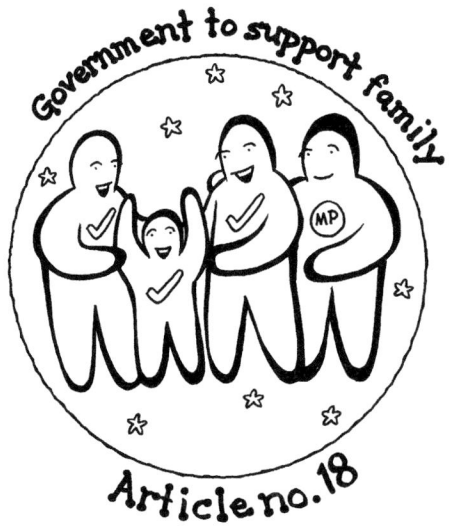

Government to support family

Article no.18

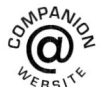

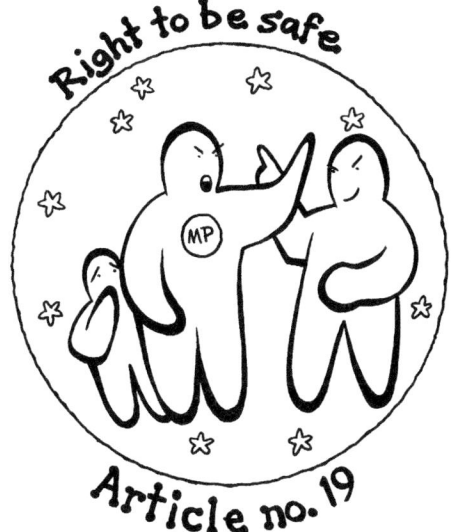

Right to be safe

Article no. 19

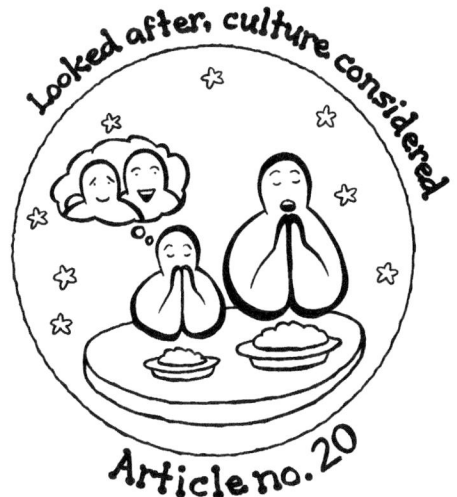

Looked after, culture considered

Article no. 20

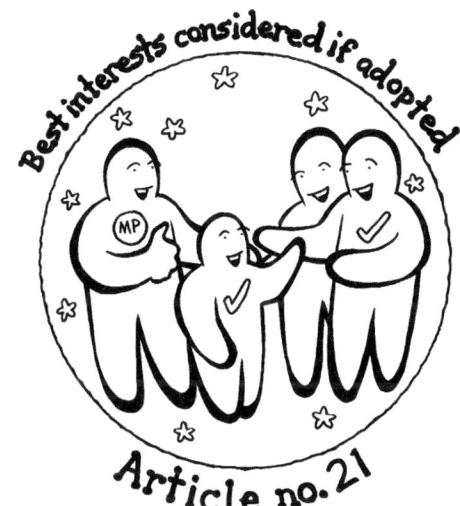

Best interests considered if adopted

Article no. 21

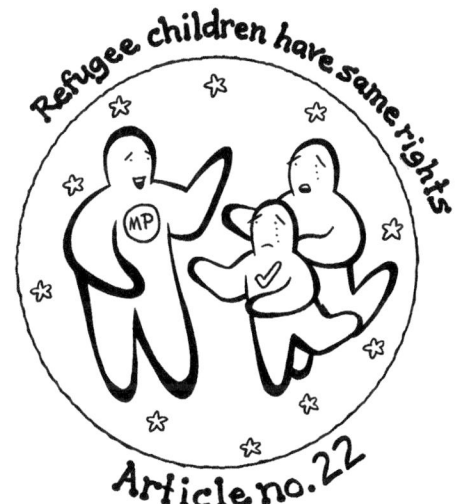

Refugee children have same rights

Article no. 22

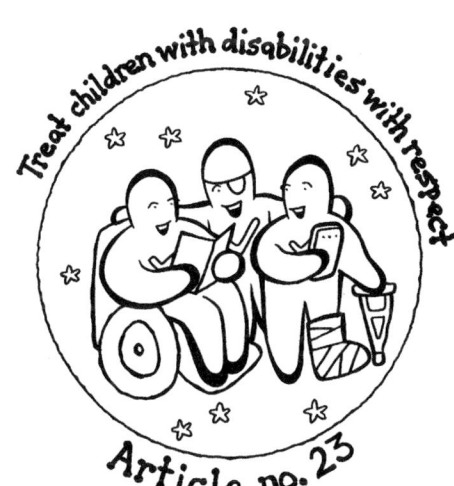

Treat children with disabilities with respect

Article no. 23

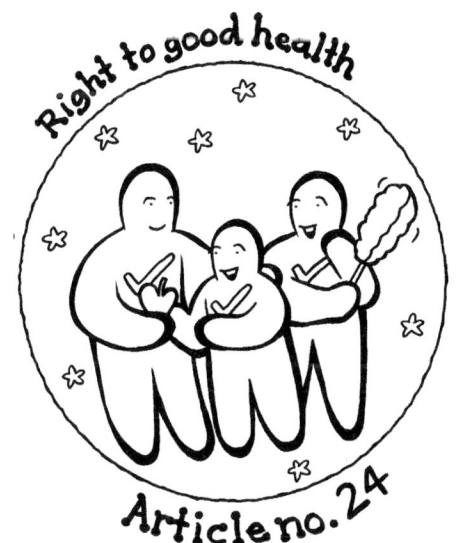

Right to good health

Article no. 24

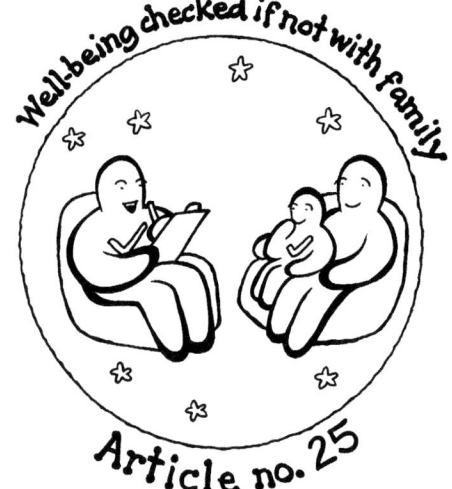

Well-being checked if not with family

Article no. 25

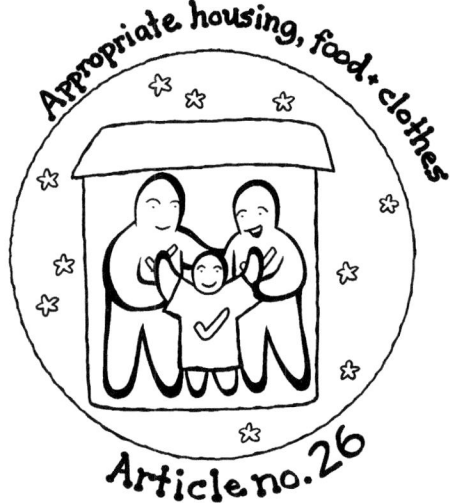

Appropriate housing, food + clothes

Article no. 26

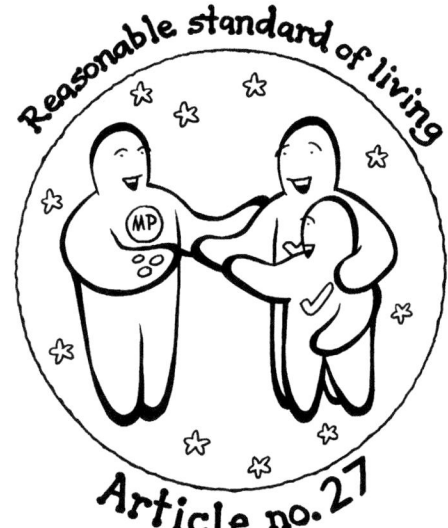

Reasonable standard of living

Article no. 27

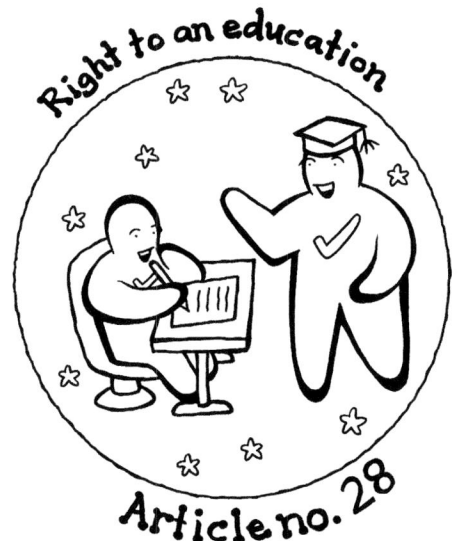

Right to an education

Article no. 28

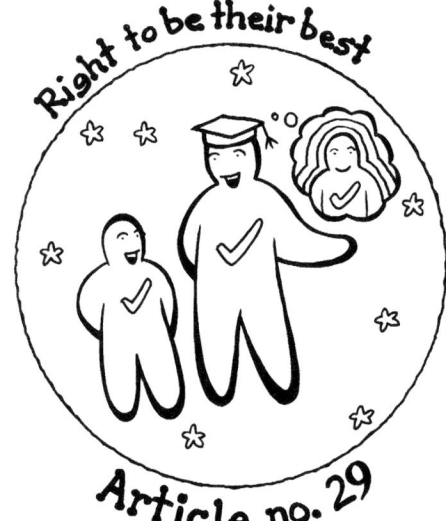

Right to be their best

Article no. 29

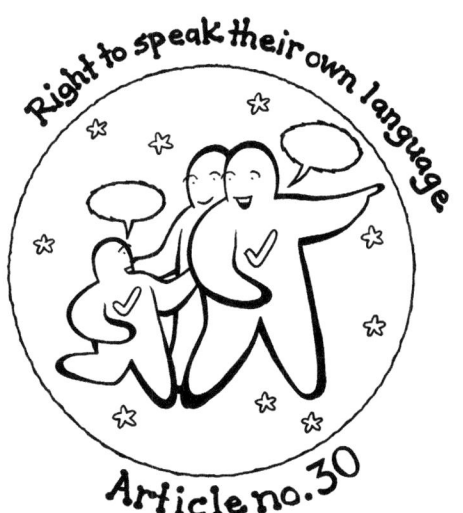

Right to speak their own language

Article no. 30

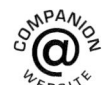

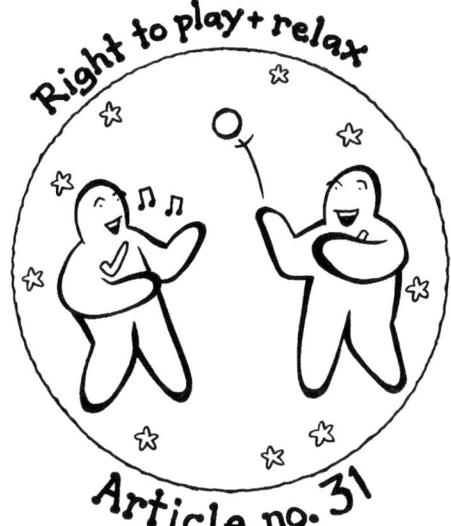

Right to play + relax

Article no. 31

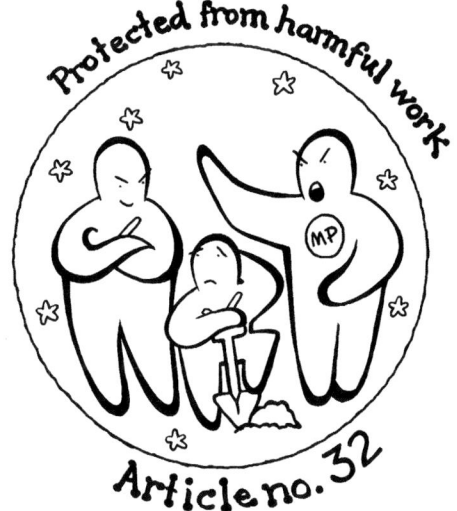

Protected from harmful work

Article no. 32

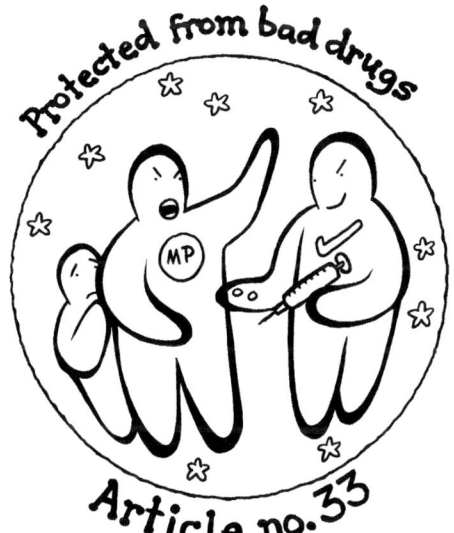

Protected from bad drugs

Article no. 33

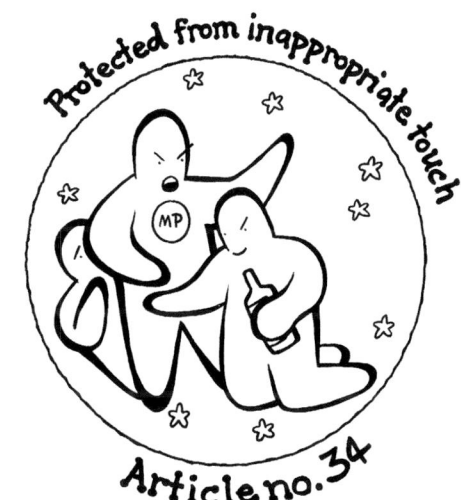

Protected from inappropriate touch

Article no. 34

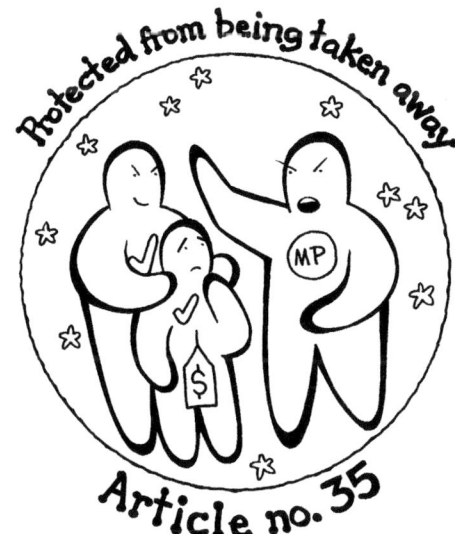

Protected from being taken away

Article no. 35

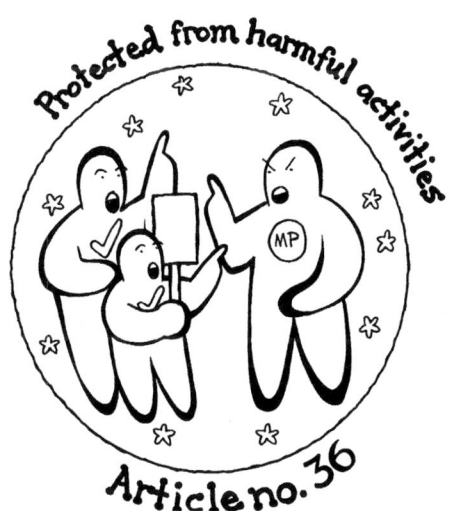

Protected from harmful activities

Article no. 36

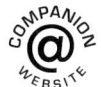

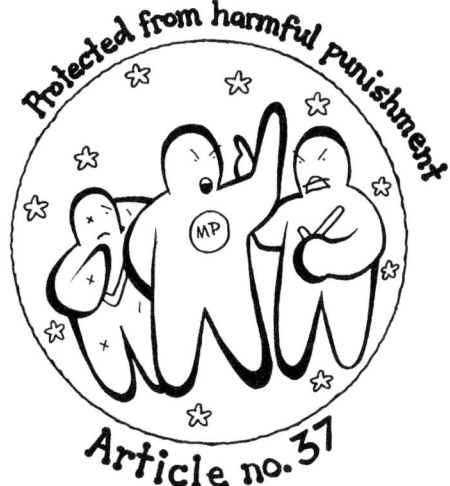

Protected from harmful punishment

Article no. 37

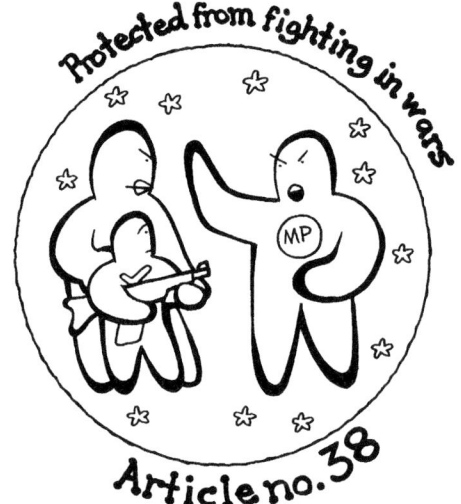

Protected from fighting in wars

Article no. 38

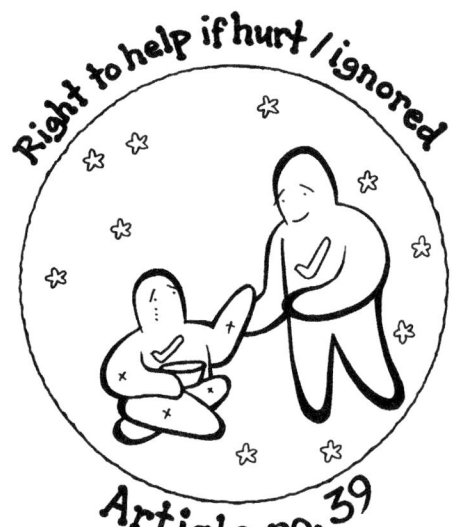

Right to help if hurt / ignored

Article no. 39

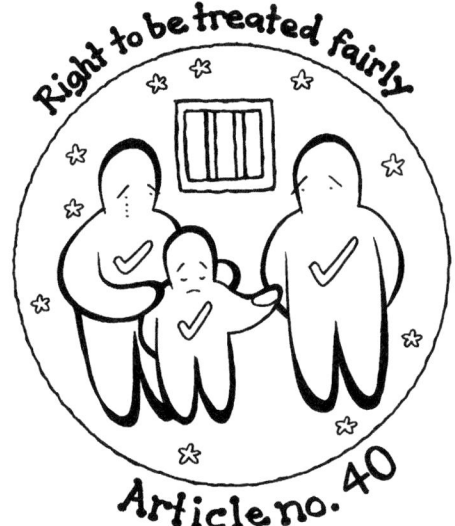

Right to be treated fairly

Article no. 40

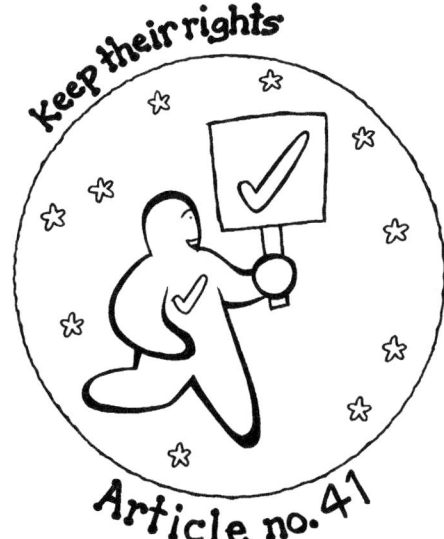

Keep their rights

Article no. 41

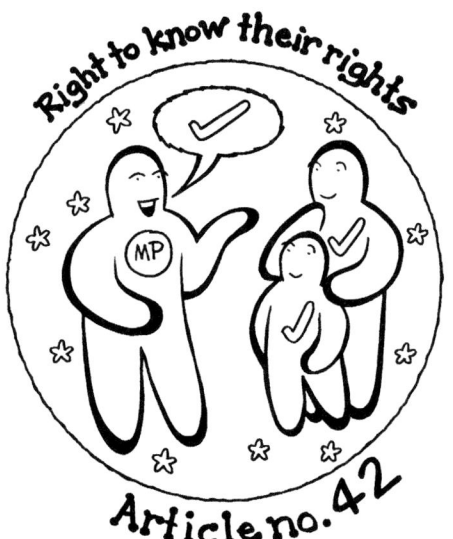

Right to know their rights

Article no. 42

Compact Blob Human Rights for Children

Hand out these sheets to your group. You may like to do one sheet at a time or all four in one go. Here are a few exercises that you might like to carry out. These can be used as quick discussion starters or be a stimulus to writing.

With your talk partner, look at all the Blobs on the sheet(s).

Which images are positive activities?

Which images are warning activities?

Which images are about being creative?

Which images are about protecting children?

Which images have MPs from the government in them?

Which images are about freedom of beliefs and religion?

Which images confuse you?

Why have the adults got ticks on their bodies as well as the children?

After each question, draw your group together and be prepared for some differences of opinion. Where these arise, turn to the written list of Children's Rights Articles in order to clarify what has been drawn.

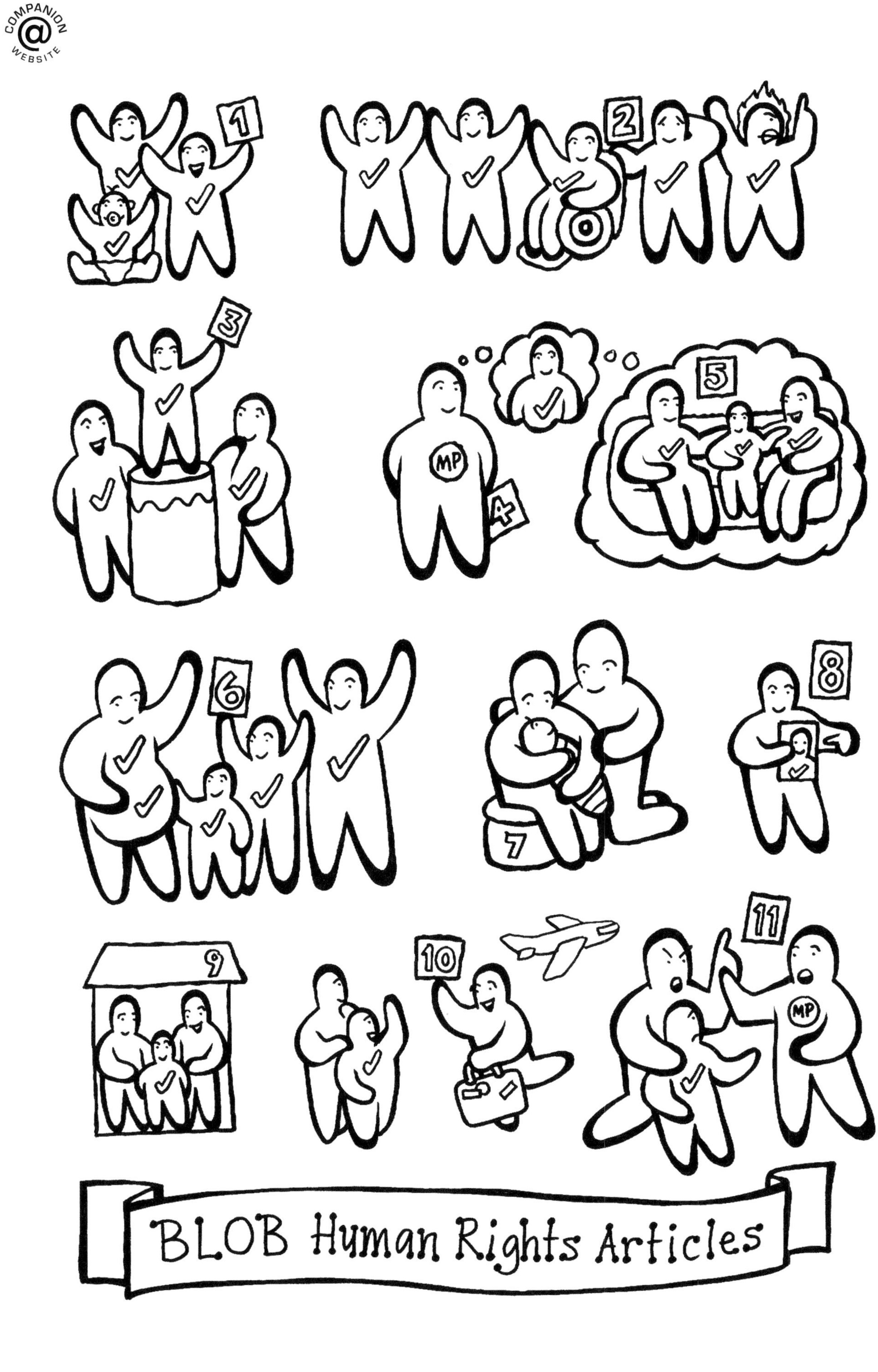

BLOB Human Rights Articles

12
13
14
15
16
17
18
MP
MP
19
20
21
MP
22
MP

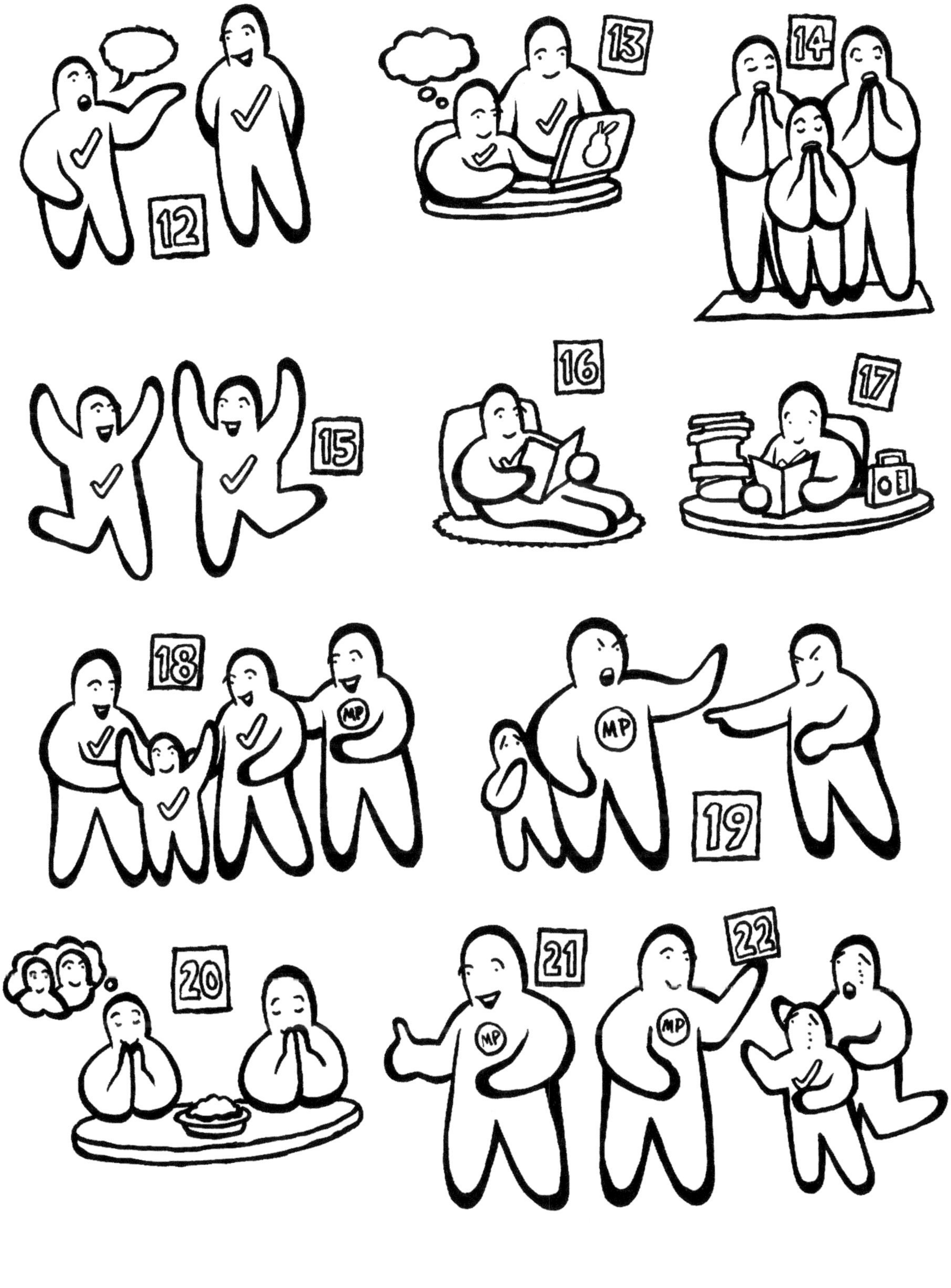

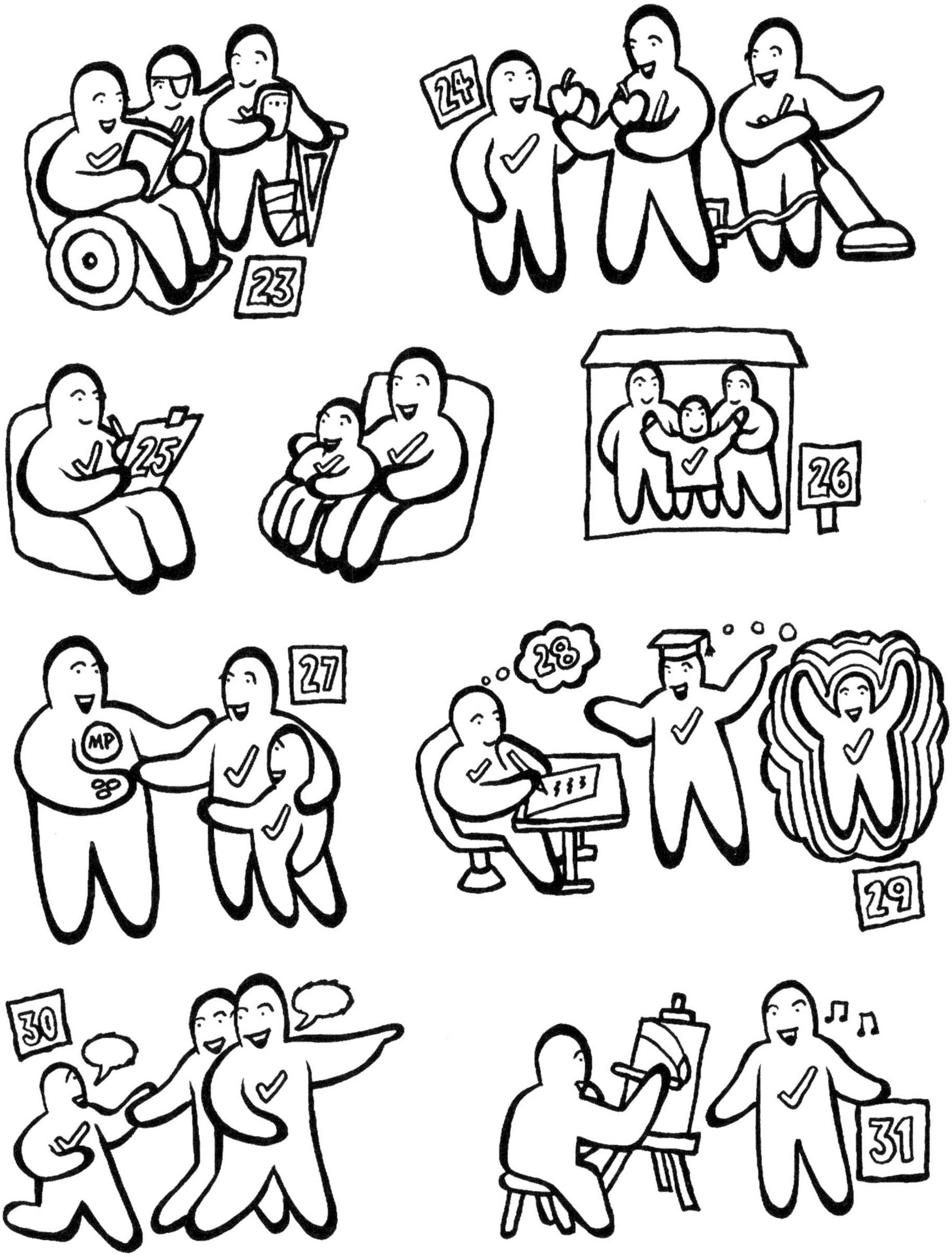

32
MP
33
MP
34
35
MP
$
36
MP
37
MP
38
MP
39
40
41
42

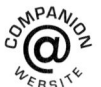

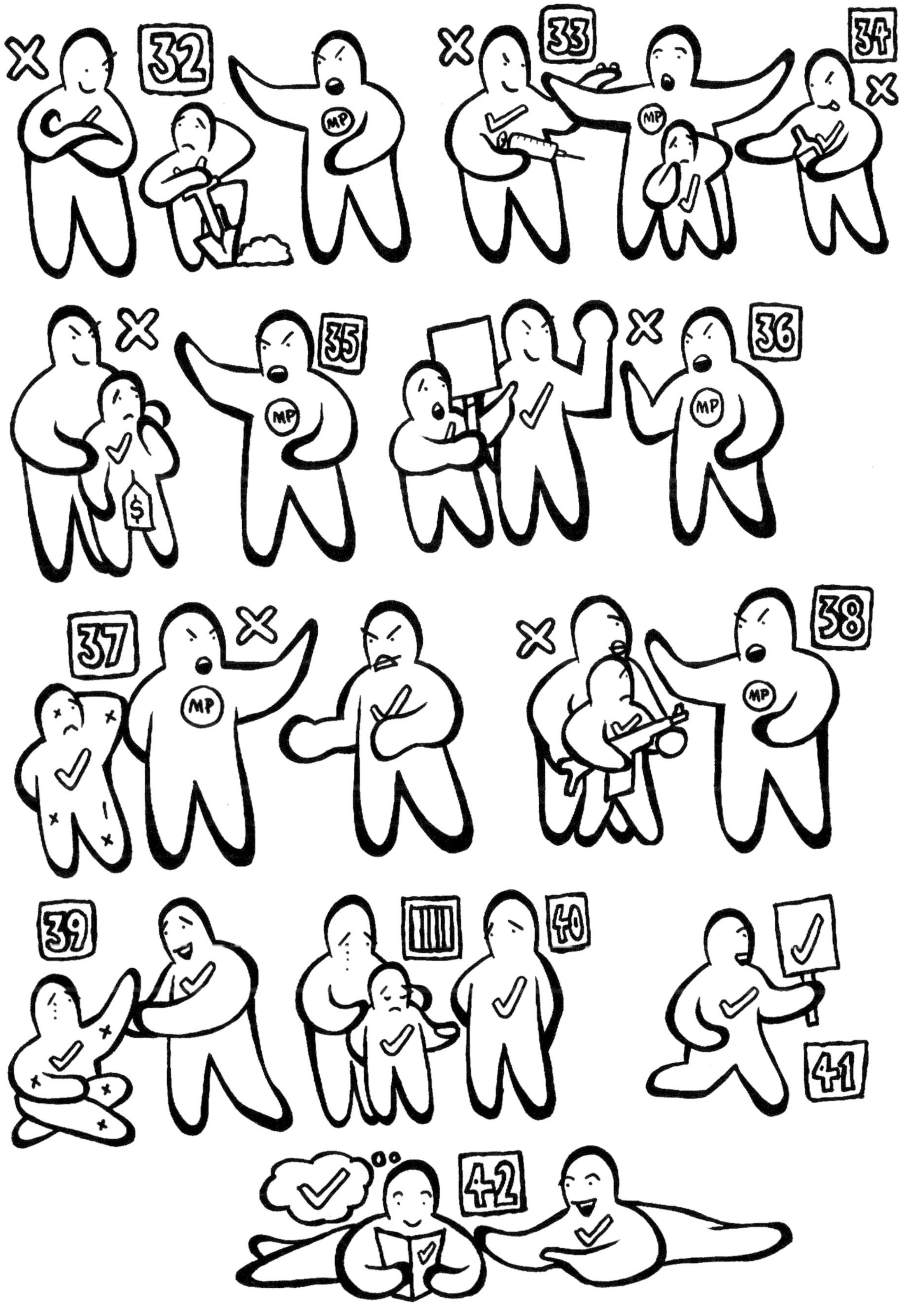

Applying Human Rights to Life

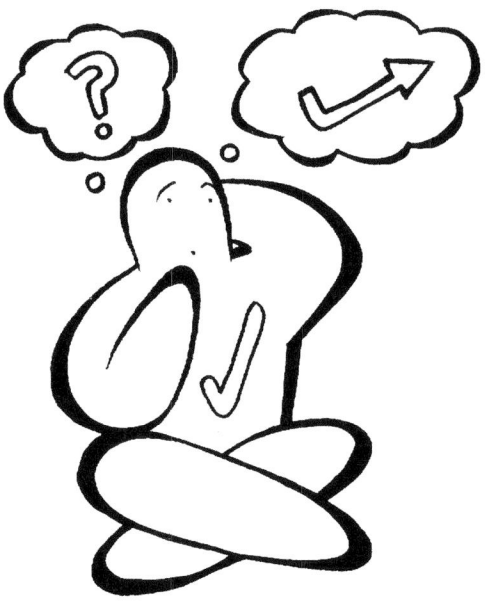

Blob We Are All Equal

The first two Children's Rights articles are as follows: Every child has the right to have rights [Article 1]; Every child has the right to equality [Article 2].

This first sheet looks at ways that some people are made to feel less equal than others.

Look at this sheet with your talk partner.

What different types of Blobs can you see?

Which Blobs would find doing some things in life difficult? Why?

Which Blobs would you find difficult to be friends with? Why?

Which Blobs have fewer human rights?

Which Blobs do you sometimes feel like?

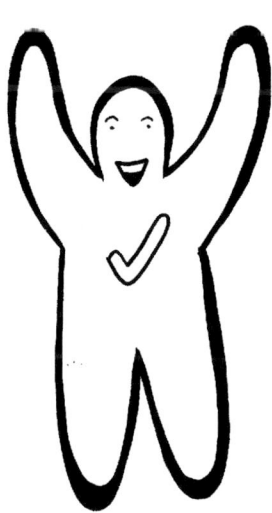

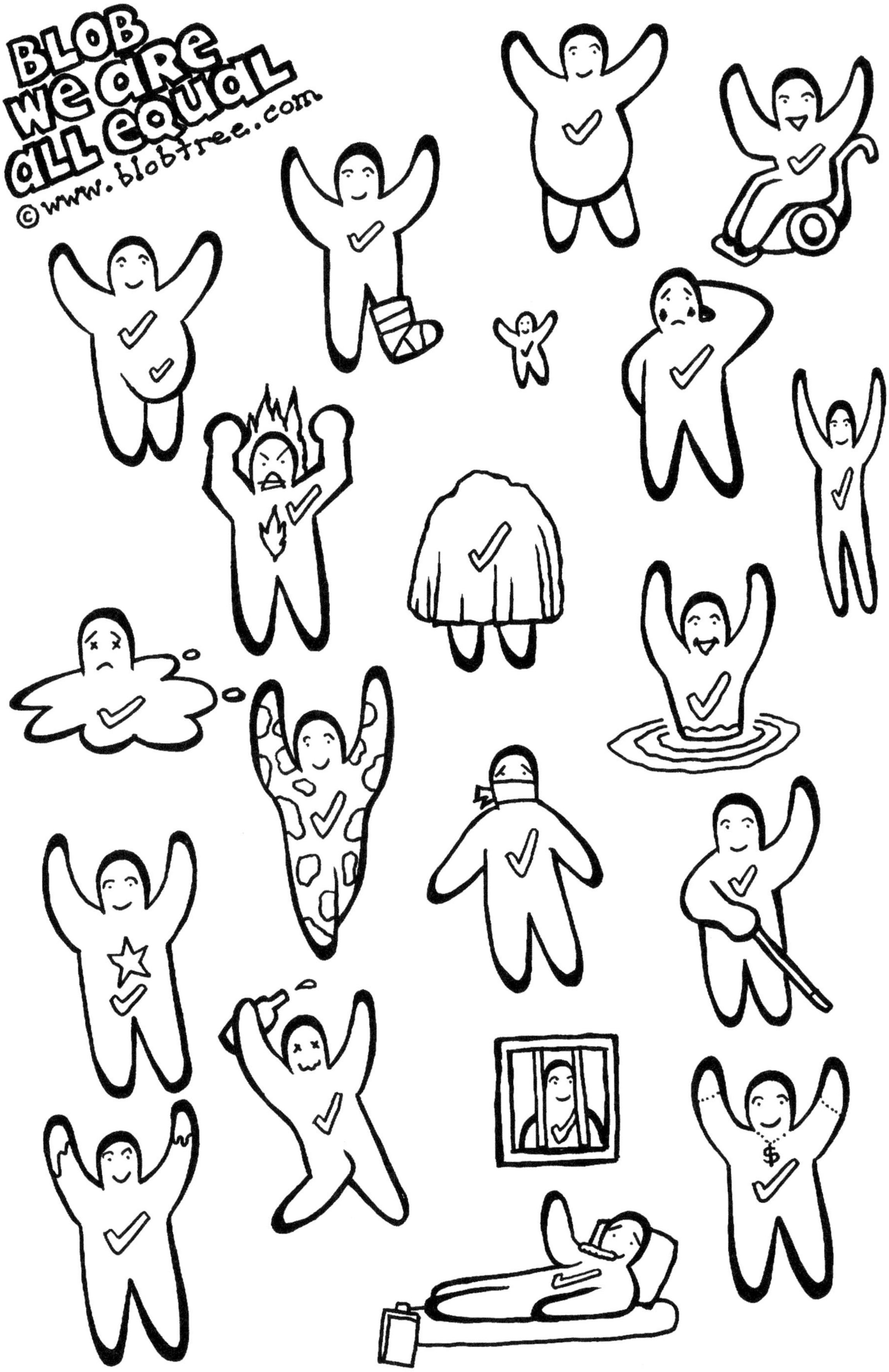

BLOB
WE ARE
ALL EQUAL
© www.blobtree.com

THE BLOB GUIDE TO
CHILDREN'S HUMAN RIGHTS

Blob Don't Discriminate

The first two Children's Rights articles are as follows: Every child has the right to have rights [Article 1]; Every child has the right to equality [Article 2].

This second sheet looks at ways that some people are treated differently by others.

Look at this sheet with your talk partner.

What different types of Blobs can you see?

Which Blobs would require more attention from doctors and nurses?

Which Blobs would require more attention from the police?

Which Blobs do you sometimes feel like?

Who do you know that treats everybody fairly like the Blob on the left?

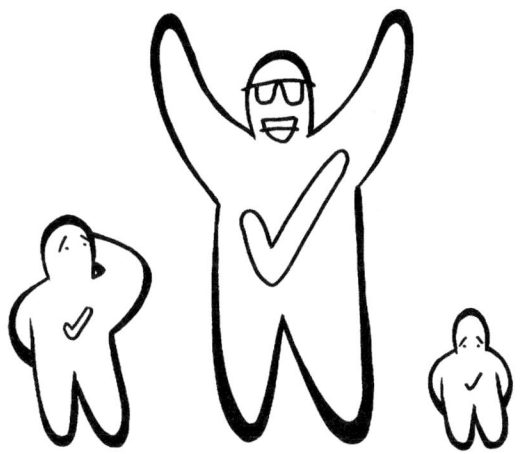

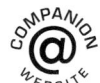

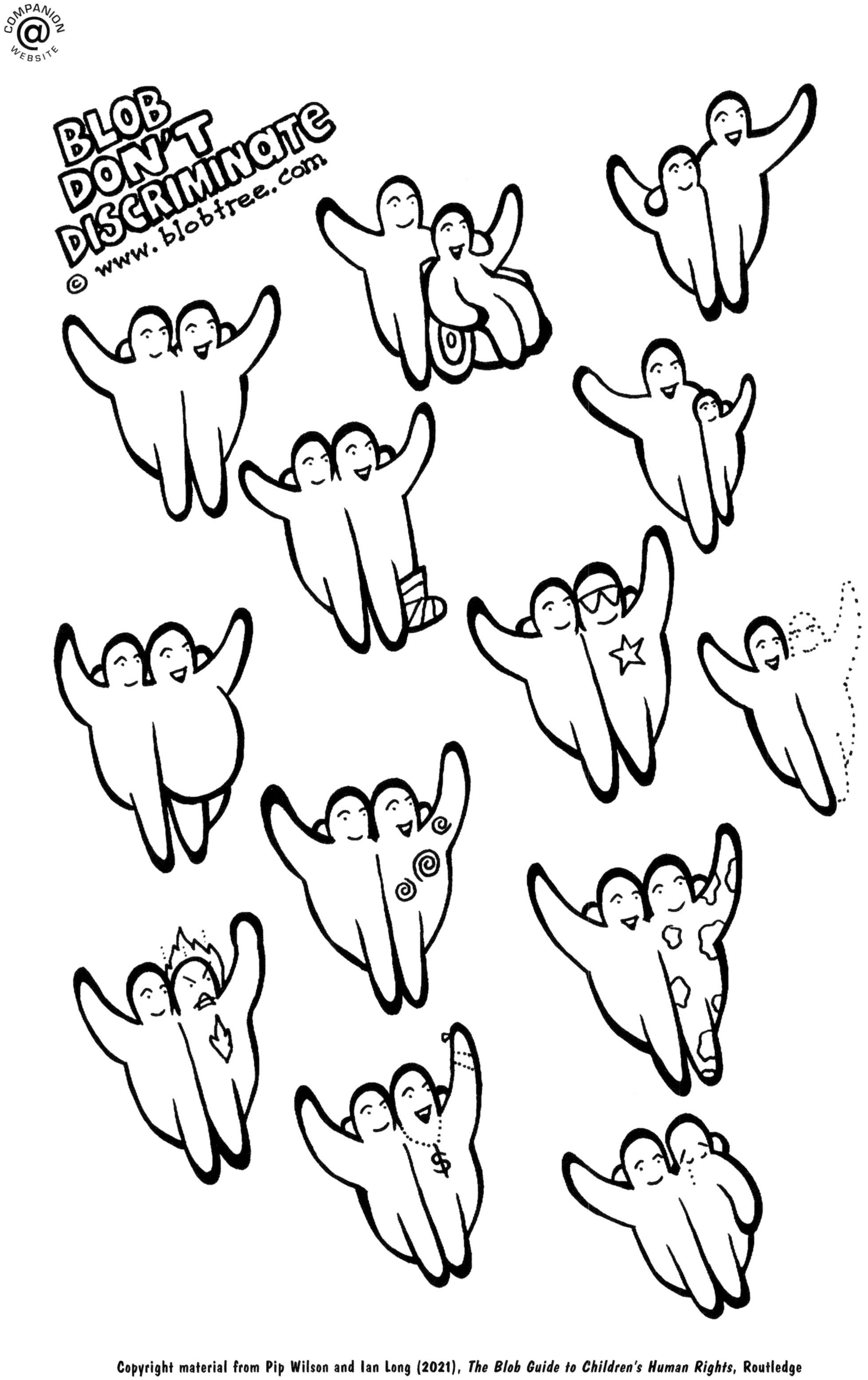

BLOB
DON'T
DISCRIMINATE
© www.blobtree.com

CHILDREN'S HUMAN RIGHTS

Blob No Rights

Imagine a world where there were no human rights for adults or children.

In some parts of the world, some people have some of their human rights removed, but imagine if they were all gone! This sheet explores some of the problems that might arise.

Look at this sheet with your talk partner.

What different types of problems can you see?

Which Blobs are having the hardest time?

Which Blobs do you sometimes feel like?

Which of these images makes you annoyed the most?

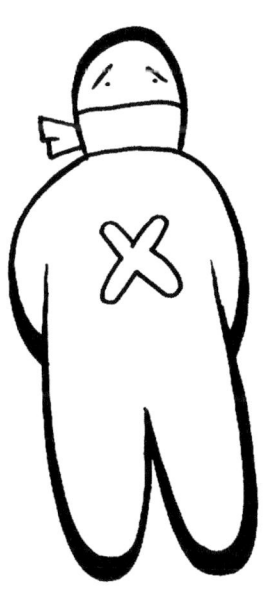

COMPANION @ WEBSITE

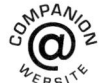

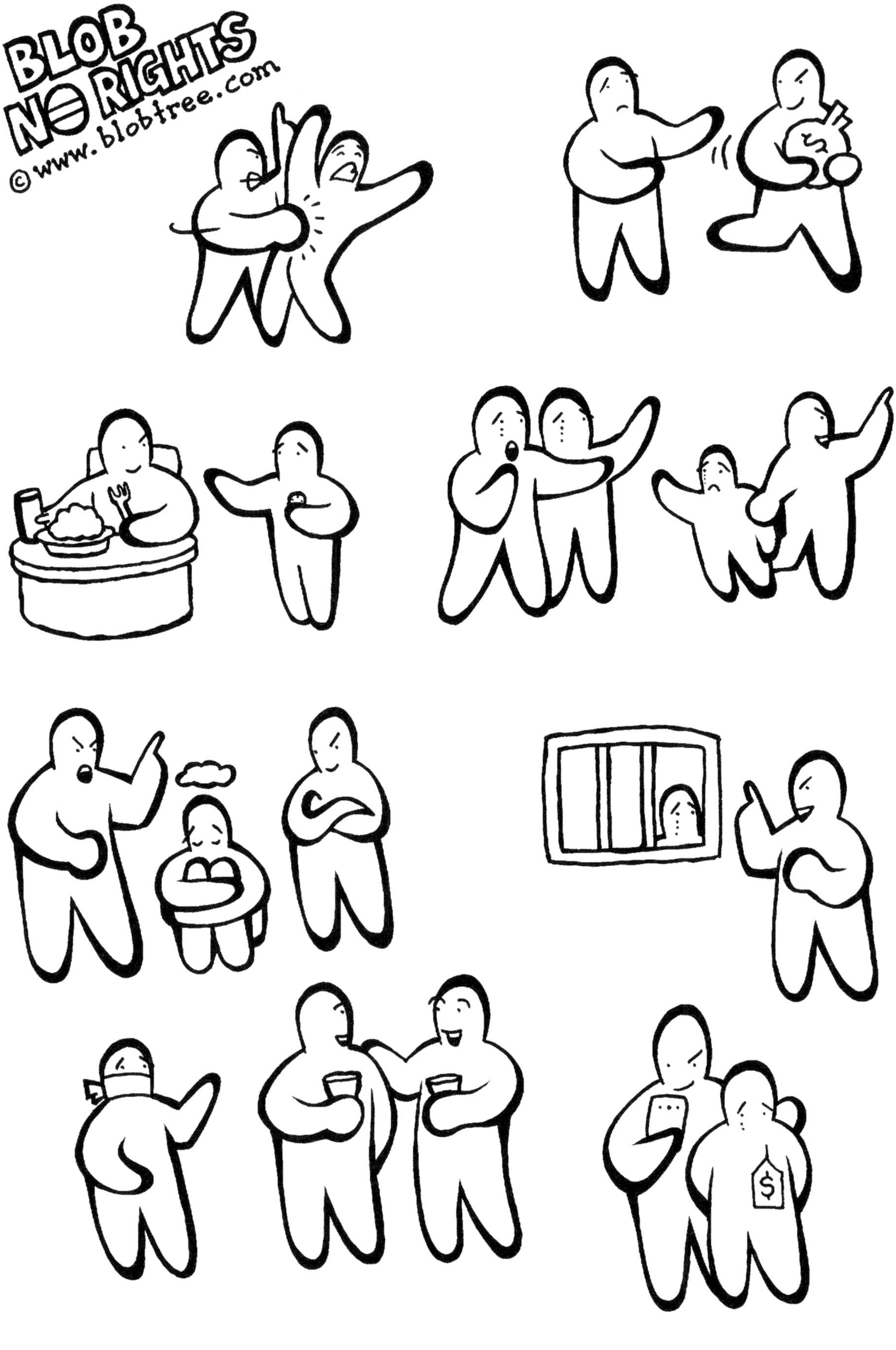

BLOB
NO RIGHTS
©www.blobtree.com

CHILDREN'S HUMAN RIGHTS

Blob Human Rights

This sheet is a quick summary of the key areas of the UN Convention on the Rights of the Child (UNCRC). As such, this sheet can be used to introduce the topic or as a simple summative assessment at the end.

Look at this sheet with your talk partner.

What different types of human rights can you see?

Which Blobs are facing the hardest struggles in your opinion? Why?

Which Blobs have you read about or seen?

Which human rights issues do you understand well?

Which human rights are the most important for you? Why?

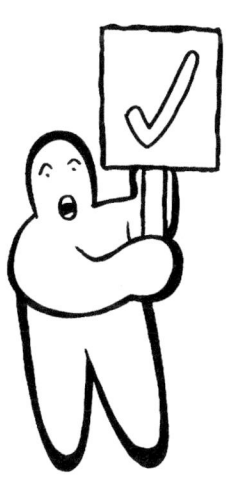

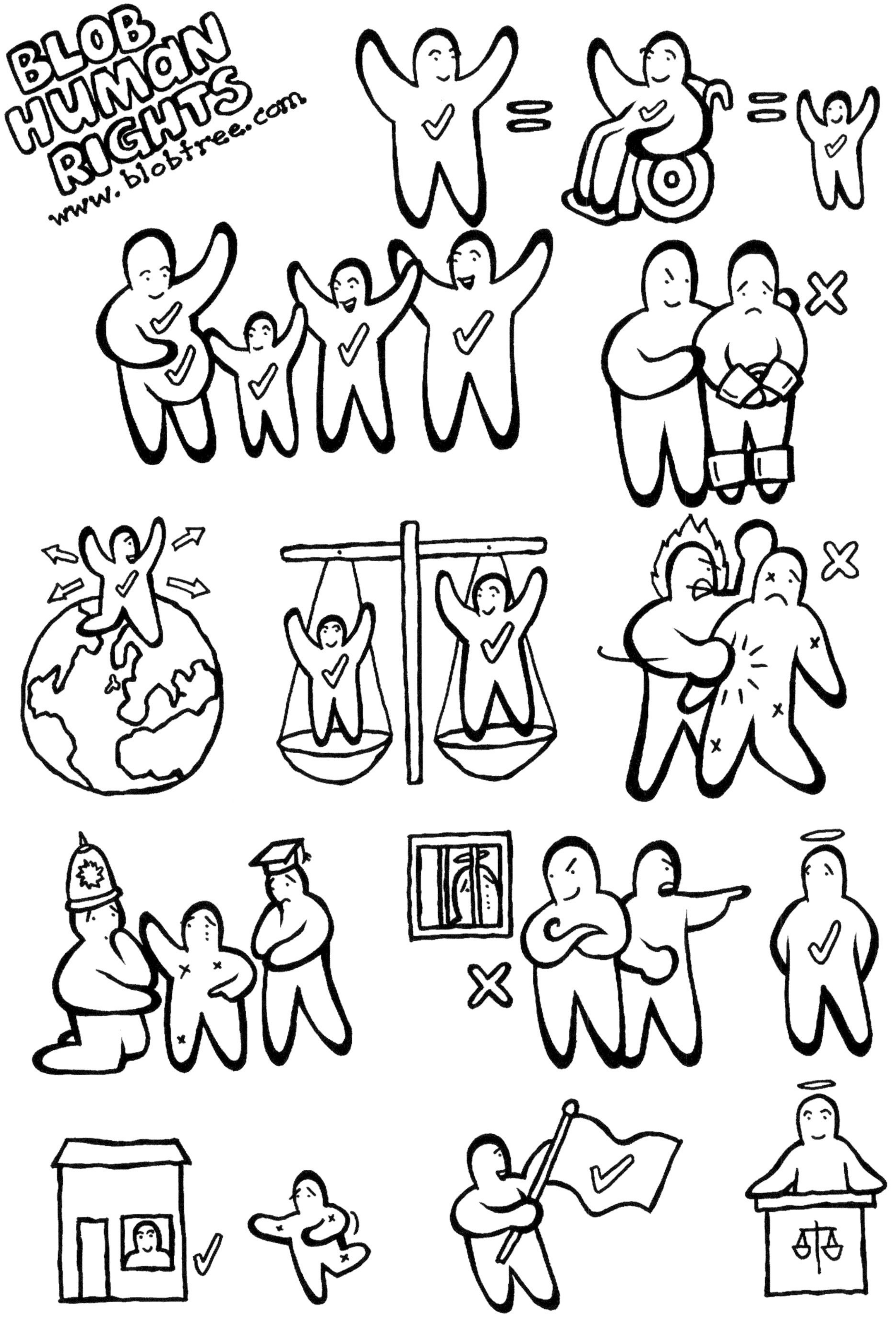

BLOB HUMAN RIGHTS
www.blobtree.com

CHILDREN'S HUMAN RIGHTS

Blob Classroom – Kind/Unkind

Every classroom tries to create a positive environment where all children can study and learn skills in a calm, affirming atmosphere. Sometimes, though, this is not the case and children and staff struggle to behave.

Look at this sheet with your talk partner.

What different types of behaviour can you see?

Which Blobs are behaving in a respectful way towards others?

Which Blobs would you find difficult to be friends with? Why?

Which human rights have been affected by the classroom behaviour? (You may need to give out a list of the forty-two Children's Rights Articles as a prompt depending on how well the children know their rights.)

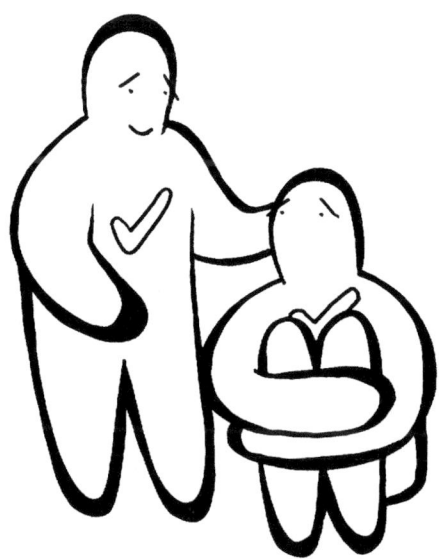

www.blobtree.com
BLOB
CLASSROOM
UN/KINDNESS
BLOB CLASSROOM

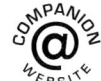

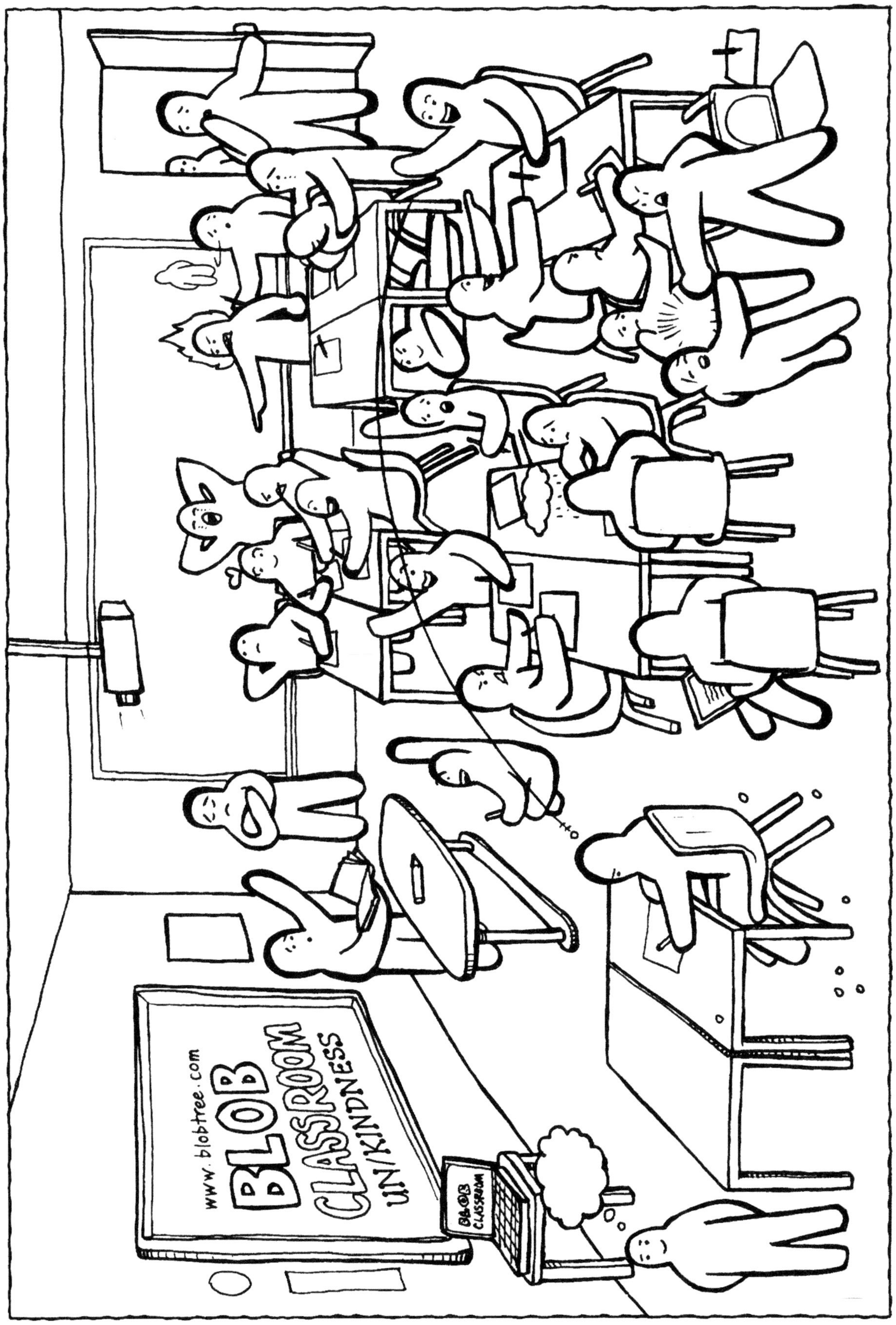

Blob Refugees

Every child has the right to the same rights as other children if they become a refugee [Article 22].

Look at this sheet with your talk partner.

What different types of Blobs can you see?

Why are Blobs looking unkindly on both sides of the water?

How are the Blobs in the boat feeling?

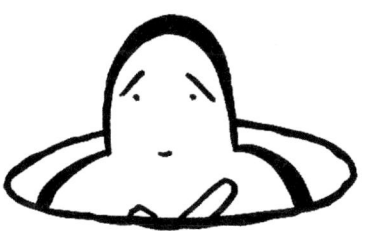

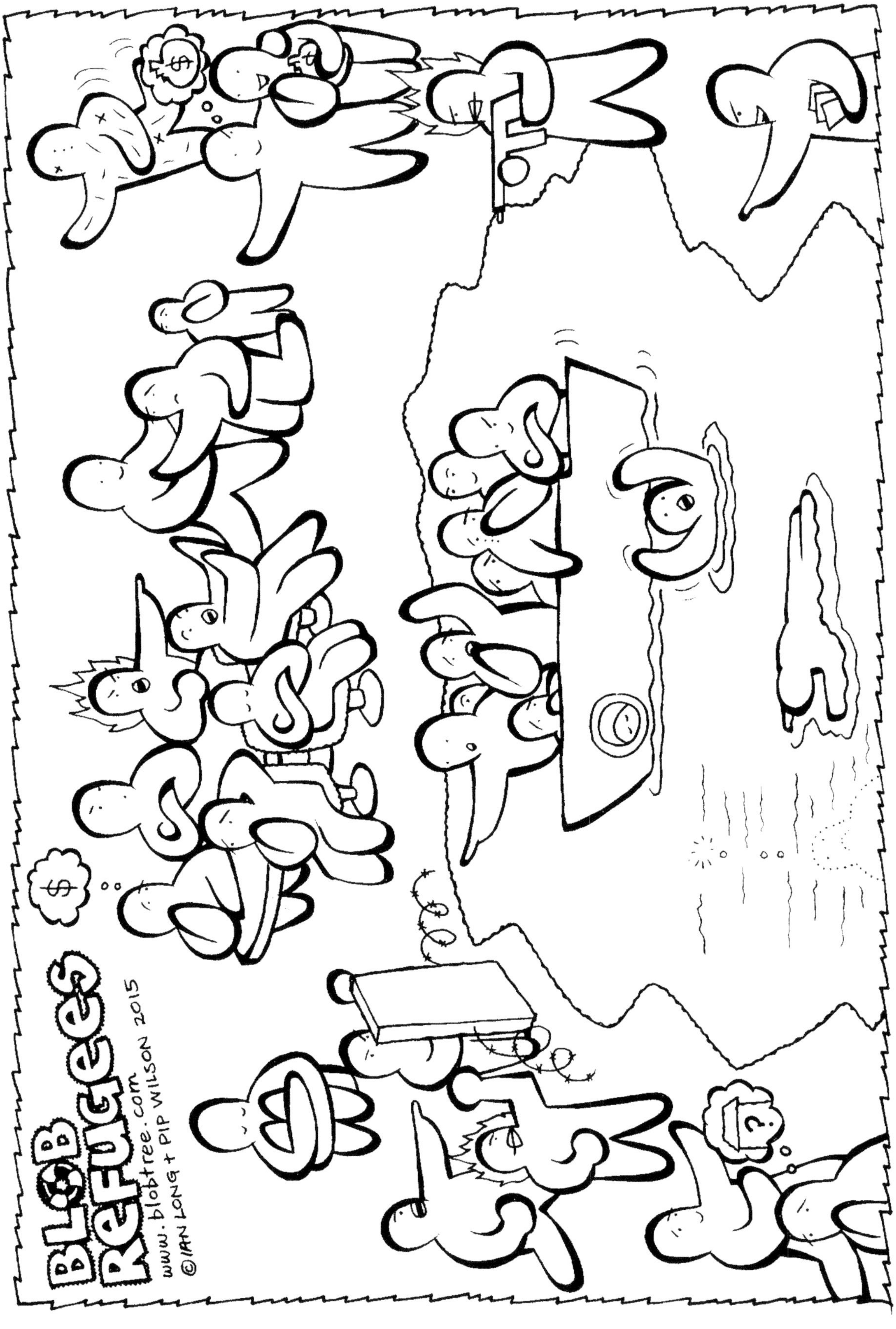

THE BLOB GUIDE TO
CHILDREN'S HUMAN RIGHTS

Blob Playground – Kind/Unkind

Every child has the right to play and relax [Article 31].

Every school tries to create a positive playground environment where all children can have fun with their classmates in a calm, affirming atmosphere. Sometimes, though, this is not the case and children and staff struggle to behave.

Look at the Unkind Playground sheet with your talk partner.

What different types of behaviour can you see?

Which Blobs are behaving in an unkind way towards others?

Which Blobs would you find difficult to be friends with? Why?

Now give out the following sheet and compare the different behaviours of the Blobs.

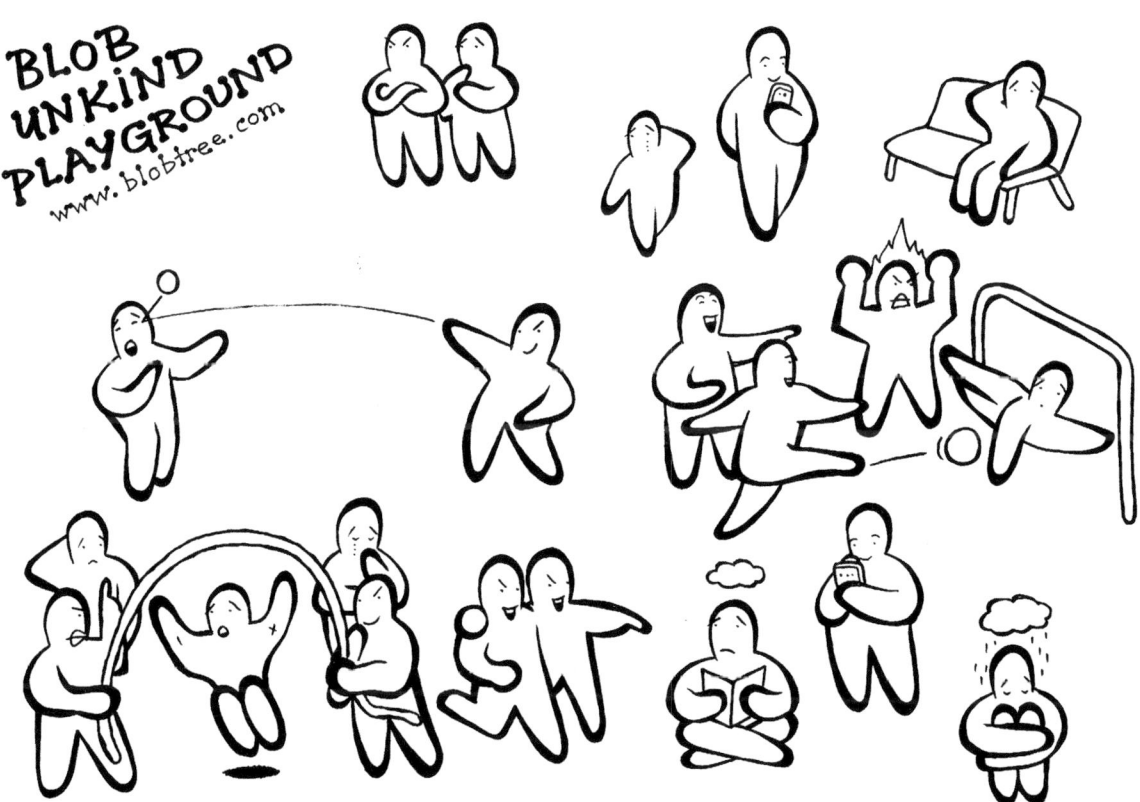

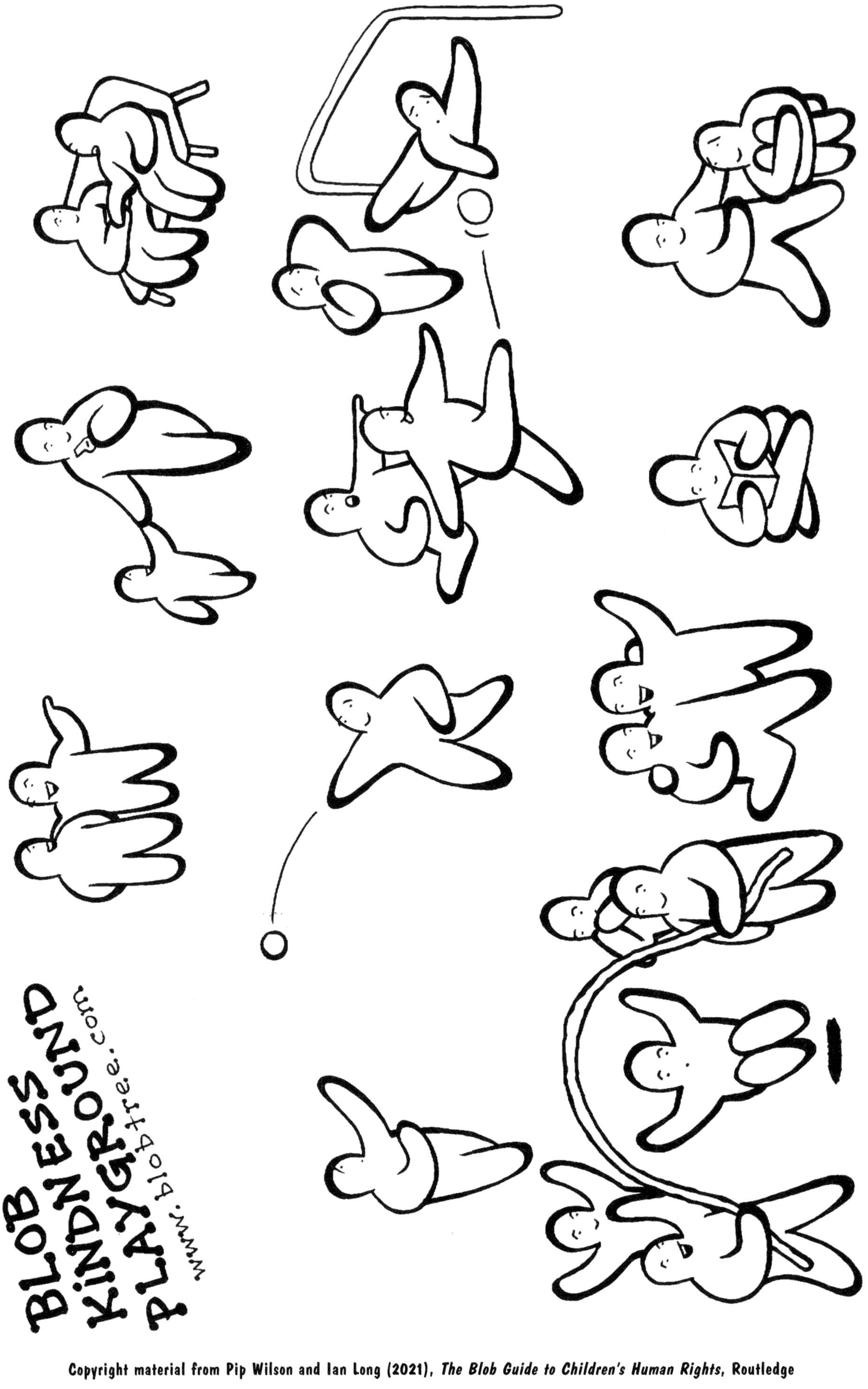

BLOB BLESS KINDNESS PLAYGROUND
www.blobtree.com

CHILDREN'S HUMAN RIGHTS

Blob Home Life

Look at this sheet with your talk partner.

What different types of behaviour can you see?

Which Blobs are behaving in an unkind way towards others?

Which Blobs remind you of some ways that you like to behave?

What human rights are being followed or being broken by these Blobs? (You may need to provide the list of forty-two Children's Rights Articles.)

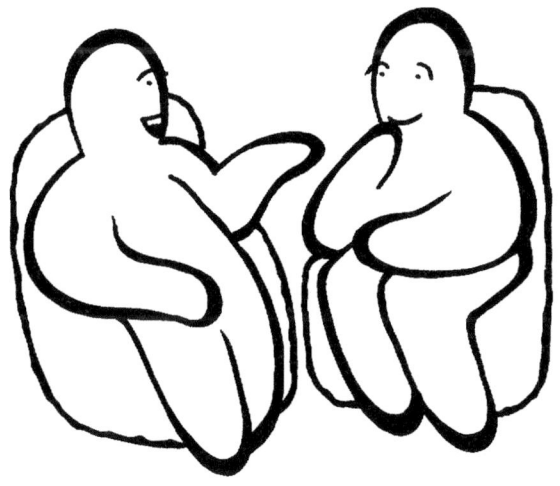

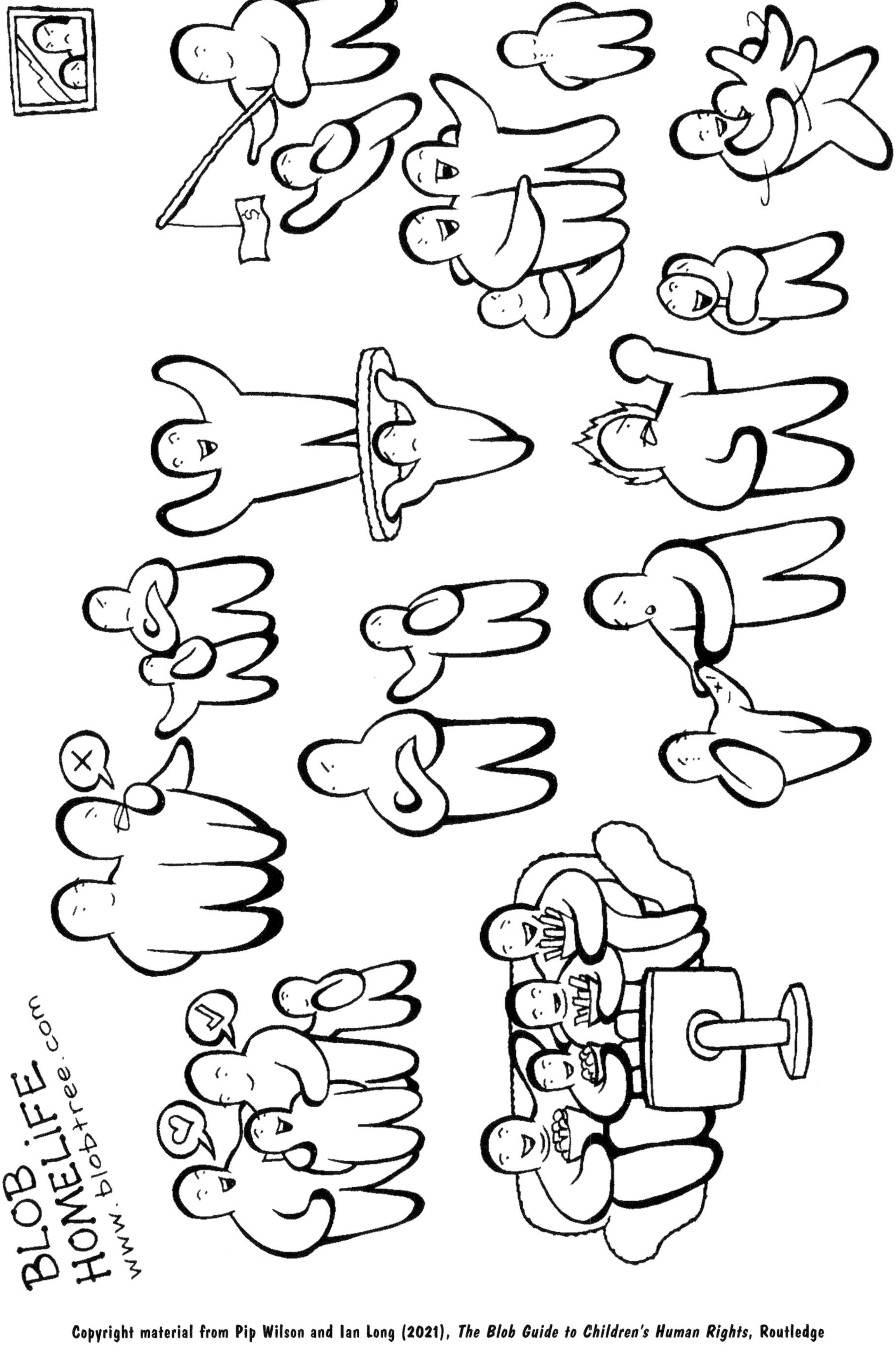

CHILDREN'S HUMAN RIGHTS

Blob Health

Look at this sheet with your talk partner.

What different types of behaviour can you see?

Which Blobs are being helpful to others?

Which Blobs are struggling to manage their own health?

What human rights are being followed or being broken by these Blobs? (You may need to provide the list of forty-two Children's Rights Articles.)

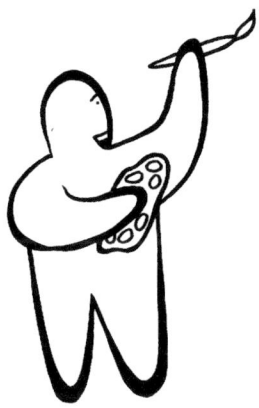

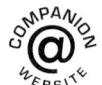

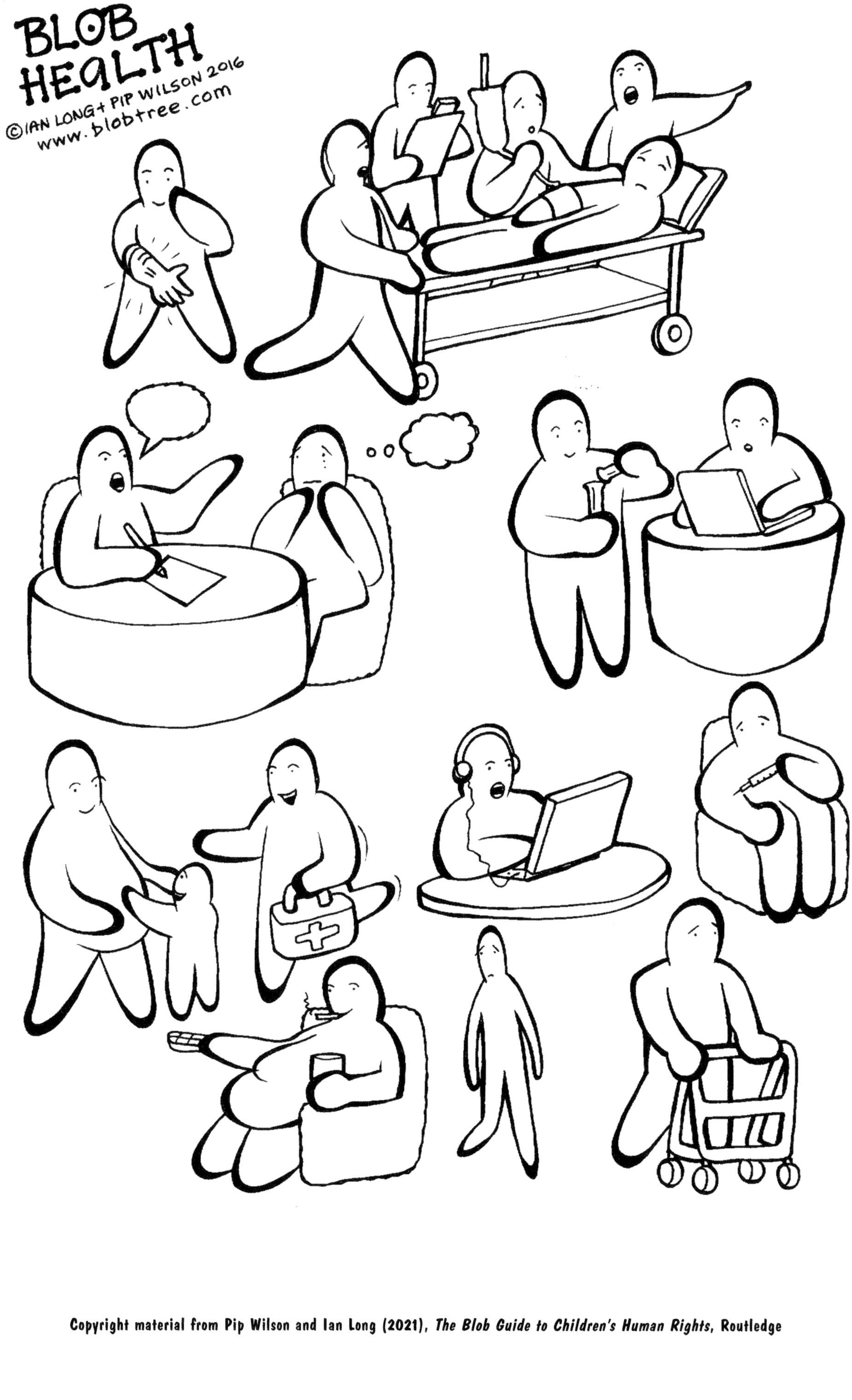

BLOB
HEALTH
©IAN LONG+PIP WILSON 2016
www.blobtree.com

Blob Trial

Every child has the right to be treated fairly if they do something wrong [Article 40].

Every child has the right to change if they do something wrong [Article 40].

Look at this sheet with your talk partner.

What different types of behaviour in trials can you see?

What are the differences between each of the trials?

Which Blobs remind you of some ways that children and adults have been treated by others when they have been caught doing something wrong?

What human rights are being followed or being broken by these Blobs? (You may need to provide the list of forty-two Children's Rights Articles.)

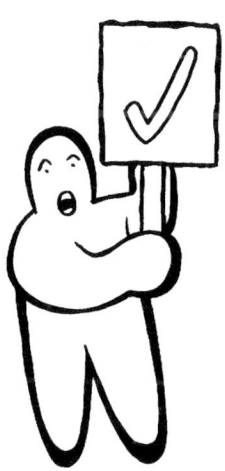

BLOB TRIALS
www.blobtree.com

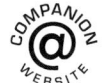

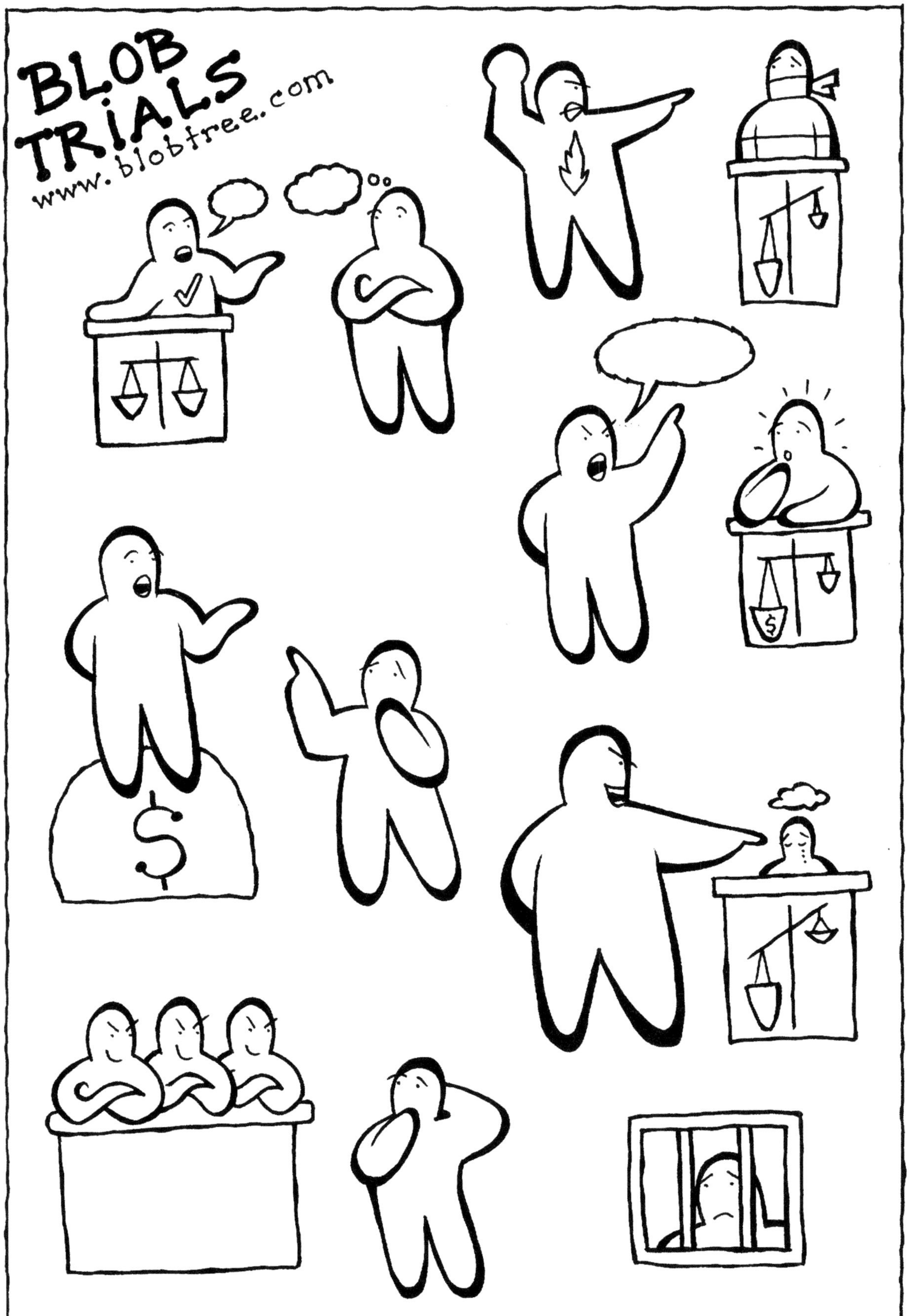

CHILDREN'S HUMAN RIGHTS

Blob Pitch

Look at this sheet with your talk partner.

What different types of behaviour on the pitch can you see?

What different feelings can you see?

Imagine this pitch represents attitudes to human rights. Those Blobs on the pitch are trying to understand and take part in human rights issues. Those Blobs in the stands are not involved. Those in the changing rooms are preparing to get involved. Those in the showers are cooling off after being involved in human rights activities.

Which Blobs have you felt like recently?

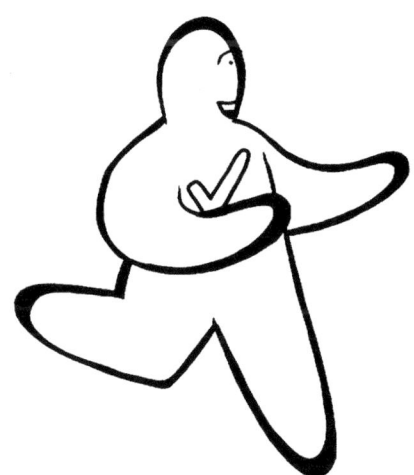

BLOB PITCH
© IAN LONG + PIP WILSON www.blobtree.com 2005

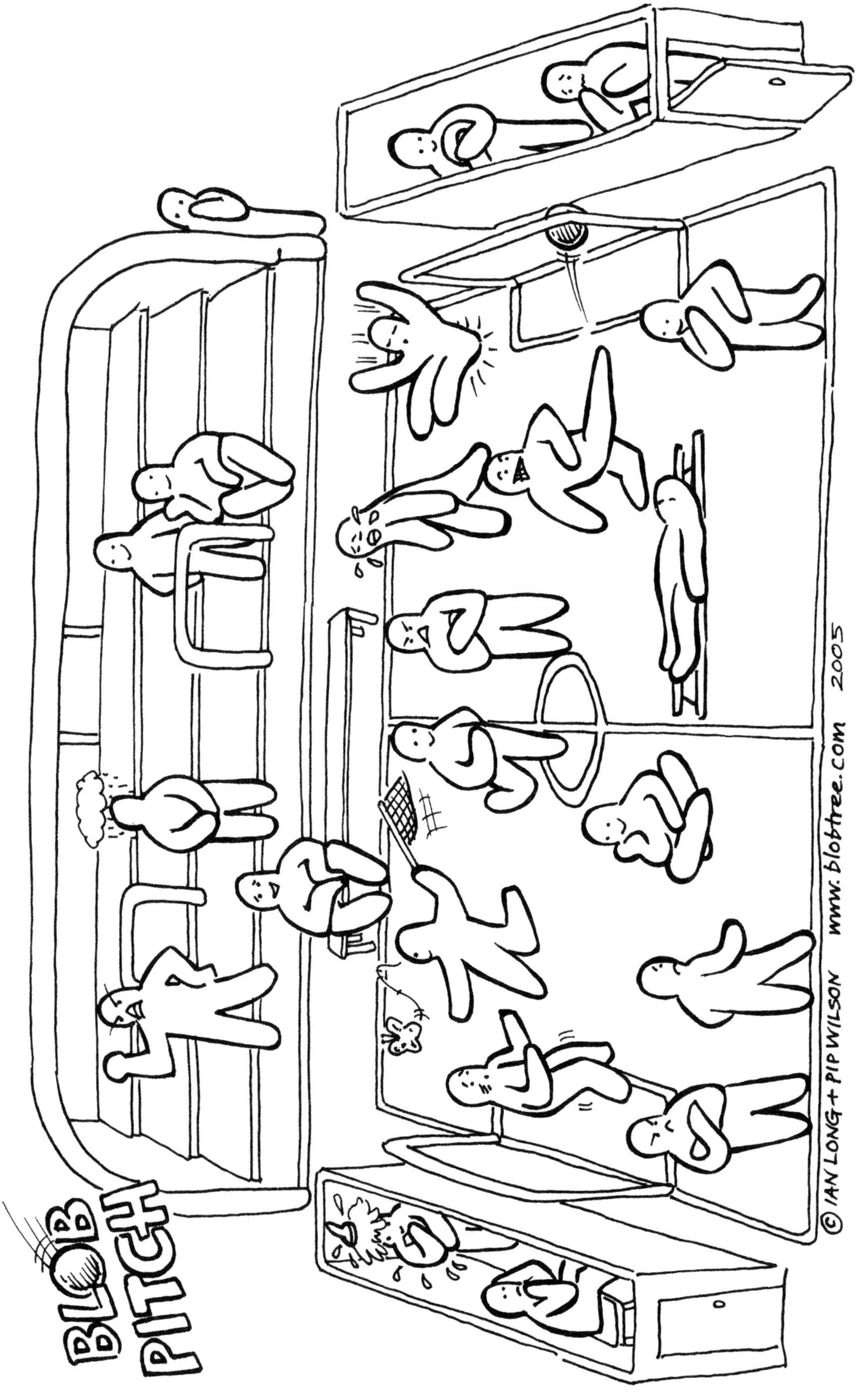

CHILDREN'S HUMAN RIGHTS

Blob Homes

Look at this sheet with your talk partner.

What different types of housing can you see?

What different feelings can you see the Blobs expressing?

Which Blobs have you felt like recently about housing?

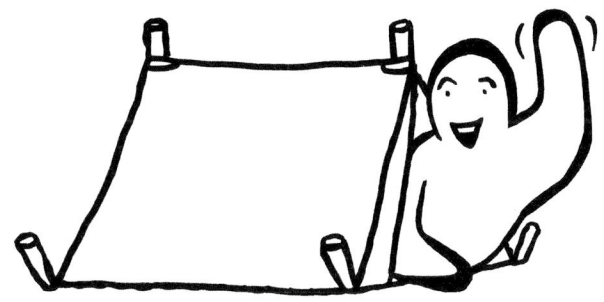

COMPANION @ WEBSITE

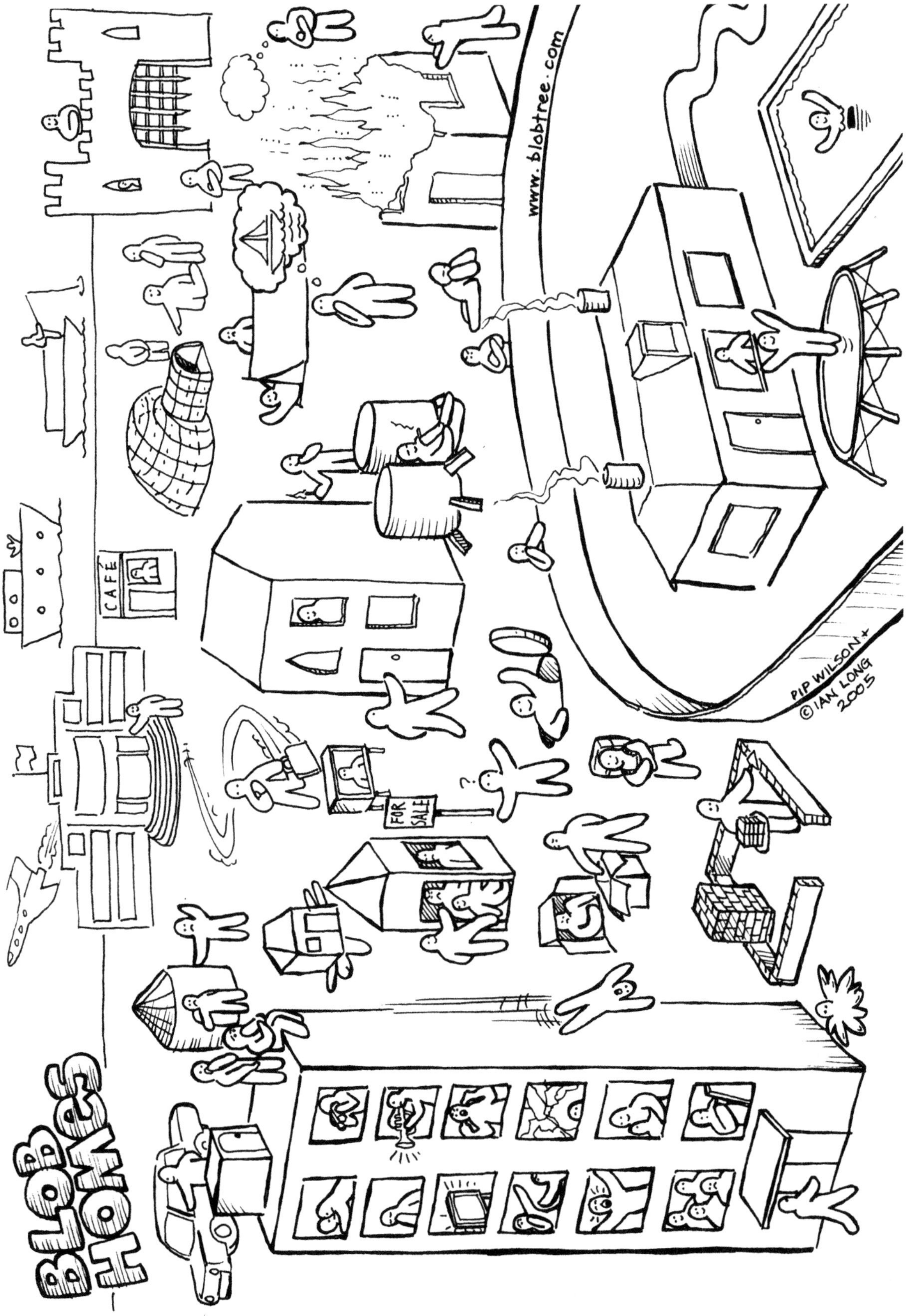
BLOB HOMES
www.blobtree.com
CAFÉ
FOR SALE
PIP WILSON + ©IAN LONG 2005

CHILDREN'S HUMAN RIGHTS

Blob Swimming

Look at this sheet with your talk partner.

What different types of behaviour around the pool can you see?

What different feelings can you see?

Imagine this pool represents how people engage with human rights. Those on the solid ground know about the idea. Those in the water are engaging with the issues.

Which Blobs have you felt like recently?

BLOB SWIMMING
www.blobtree.com
© IAN LONG 2005 + PIP WILSON

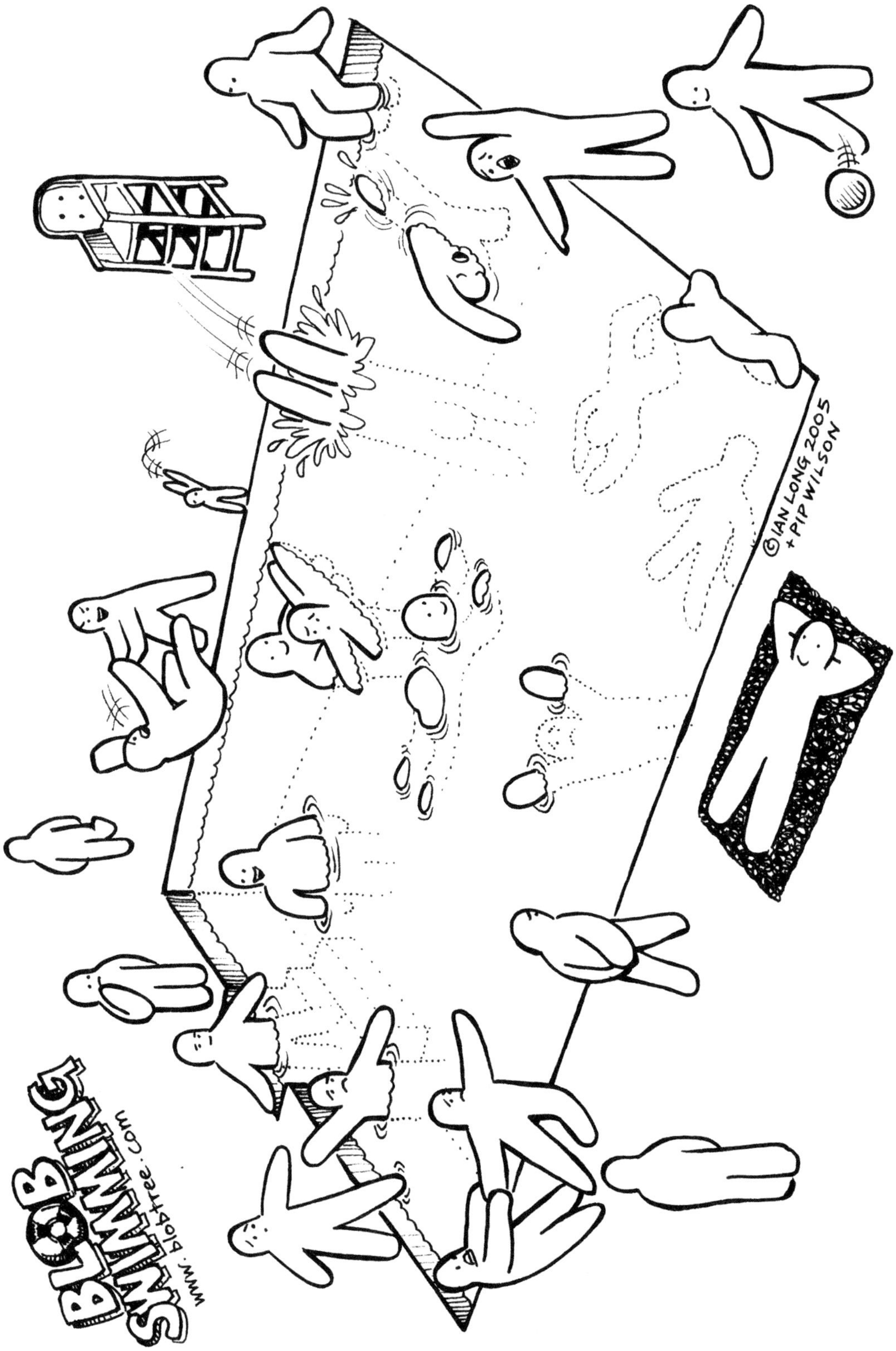

CHILDREN'S HUMAN RIGHTS

Blob Human Rights Hierarchy?

Look at this sheet with your talk partner.

What can you see that is different between the Blobs?

What different feelings can you see?

The UN Convention on the Rights of the Child (UNCRC) was written because it was believed that all people are equal and should be treated the same. Why do you think some people get treated differently in the world?

If you were to redraw this diagram, so that all people were treated equally, what would have to change?

Which Blobs have you felt like recently?

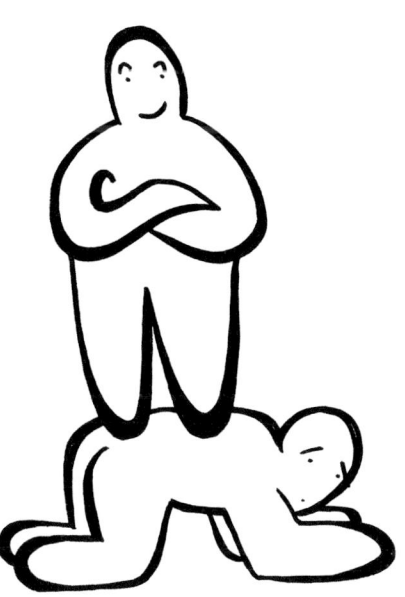

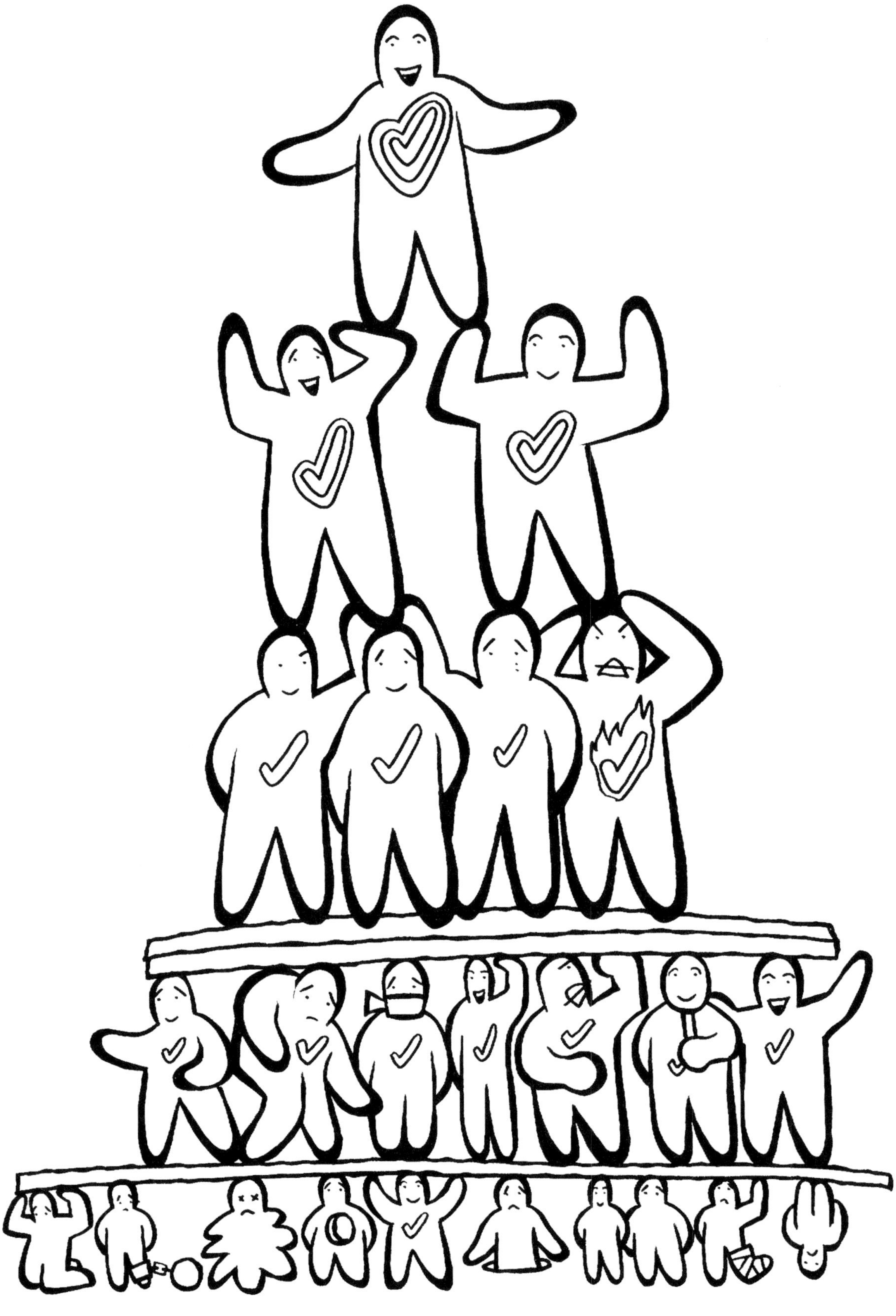

Blob World Sheets

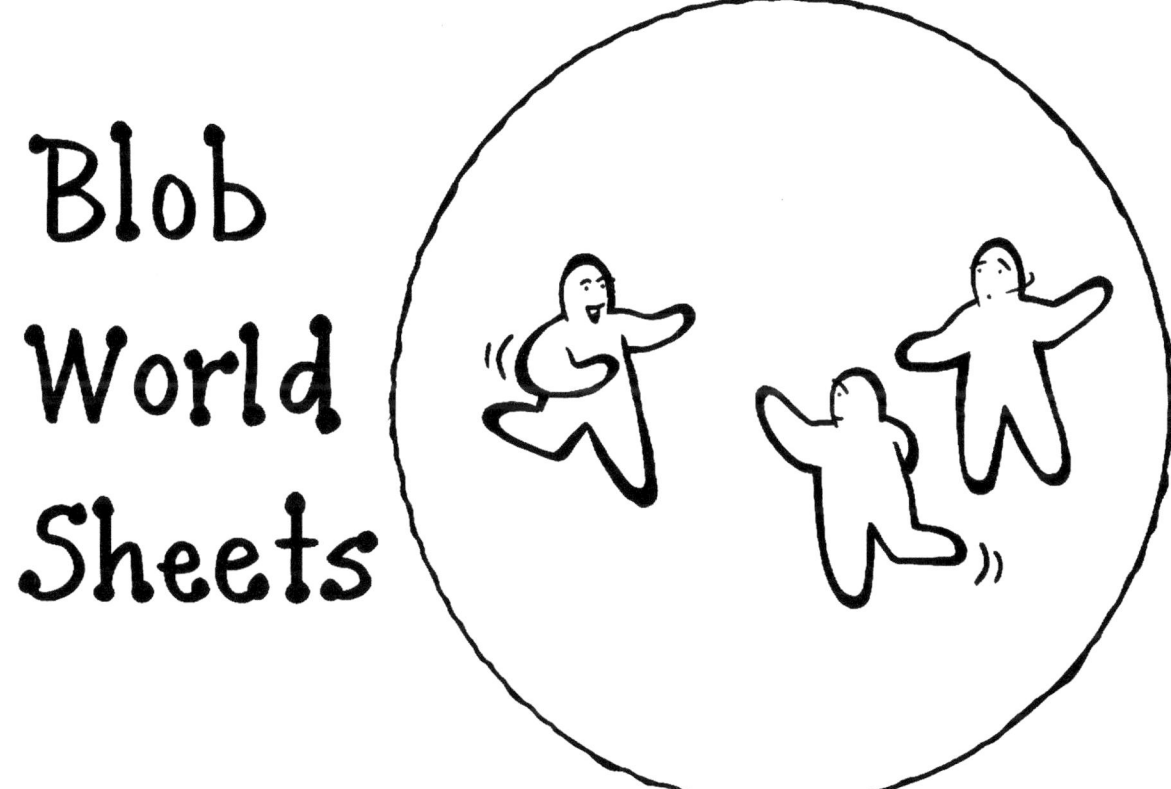

CHILDREN'S HUMAN RIGHTS

Blob World

Look at this sheet with your talk partner. It focuses primarily upon the way that we treat the world and one another.

What are the different ways that the Blobs are treating the world?

What are the different ways that the Blobs are treating one another?

Which Blob(s) have you felt like?

What human rights are being followed or being broken by these Blobs? (You may need to provide the list of forty-two Children's Rights Articles.)

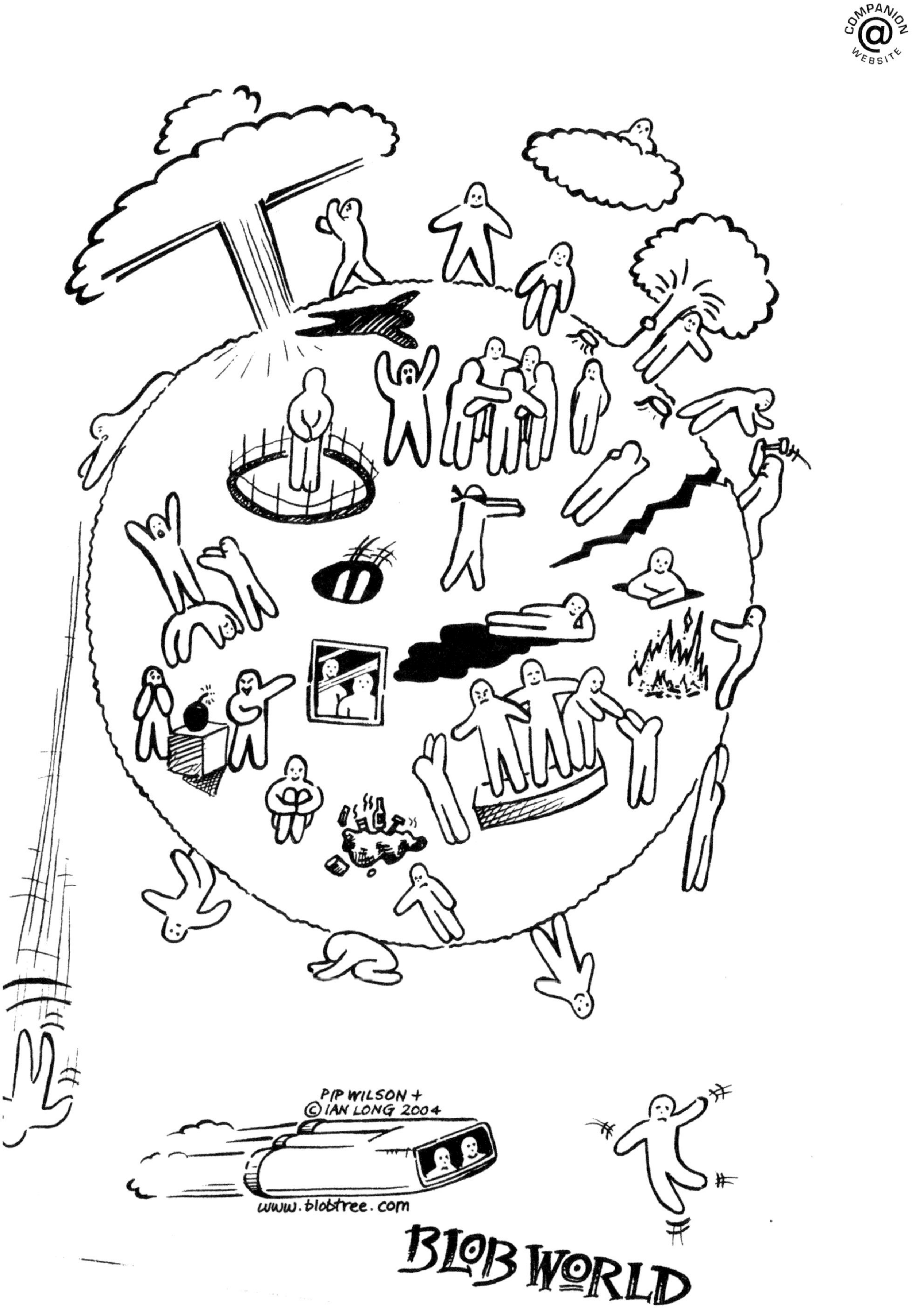

PIP WILSON +
©IAN LONG 2004

www.blobtree.com

BLOB WORLD

Blob World 2

Look at this sheet with your talk partner.

What is happening in this world?

What feelings words could you give to the Blobs at the top and the Blobs at the bottom?

Why do you think that things won't change in this world?

What human rights are being followed or being broken by these Blobs? (You may need to provide the list of forty-two Children's Rights Articles.)

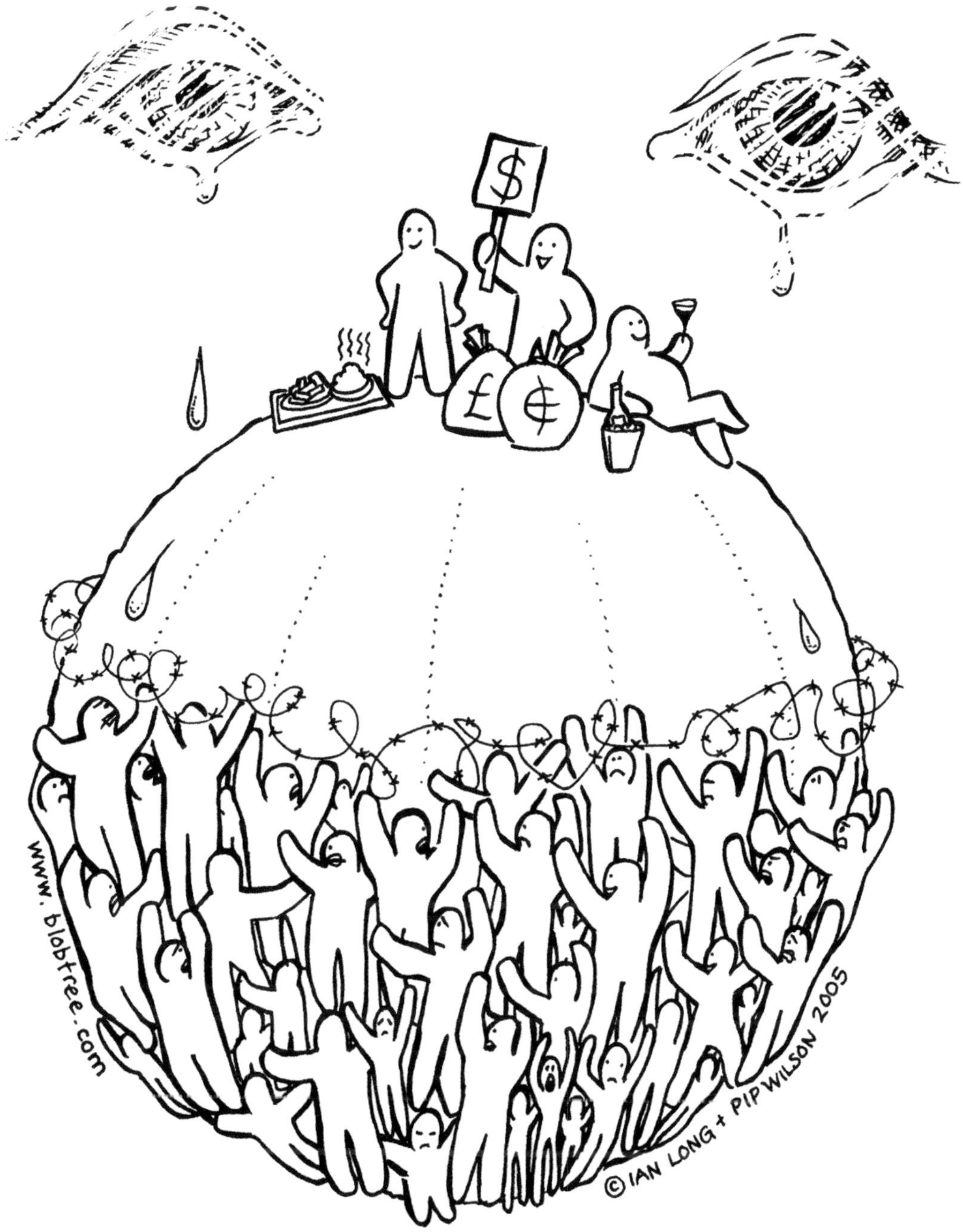

BLOB WORLD 2

CHILDREN'S HUMAN RIGHTS

Blob Two Worlds

Look at this sheet with your talk partner.

What is happening in these two worlds?

What feelings words could you give to the Blobs in the left-hand world and the Blobs in the right-hand world?

What could happen to change the differences between these worlds?

If you were a Blob in the left-hand world, what could you do to make positive change?

What human rights are being followed or being broken by these Blobs? (You may need to provide the list of forty-two Children's Rights Articles.)

Blob Two Worlds

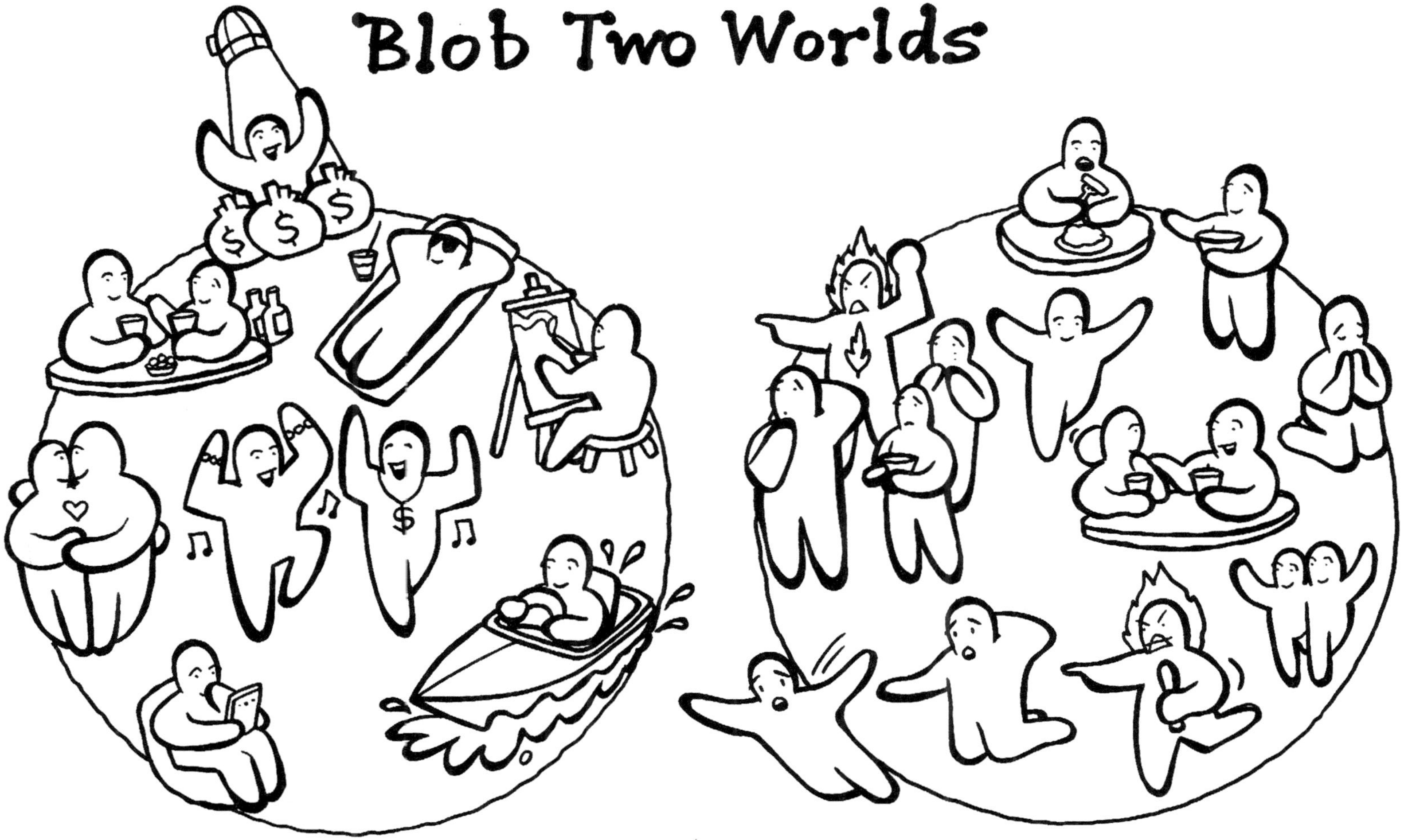

www.blobtree.com

Blob
Priority
Sheets

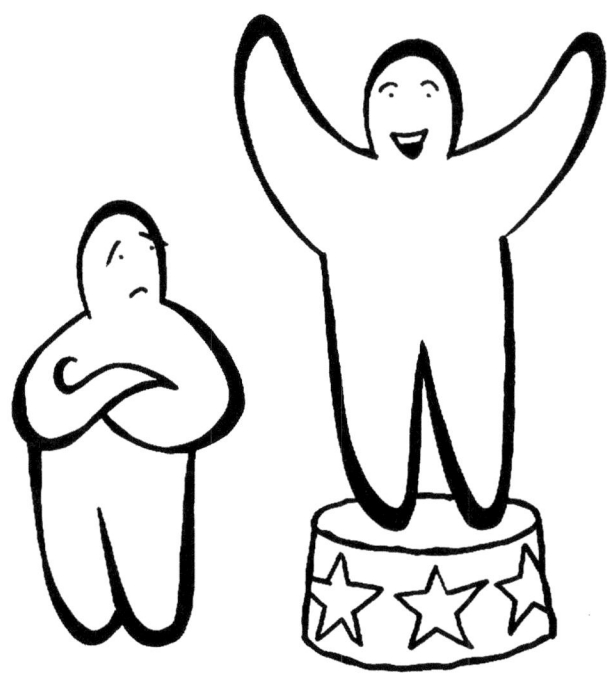

CHILDREN'S HUMAN RIGHTS

Blob Priority Sheets

Prioritising human rights issues, the elements of a day or our individual needs helps us to reflect upon how we make choices, and sharing that with others reveals how different we all are.

The next two pages show different ways of sorting the human rights images.

The **first grid** is a 3 × 4 grid which can be used to sort a larger group of images (e.g. Human Rights, Needs, Needs and Wants) in a variety of ways. For example:

Select twelve images out of a larger group of images.

With the grid in portrait orientation, place the most important elements in the top row, the second three in the second, etc.

This can be modified by having it as above but making the image on the left of each row the most important and the image on the right of each row the least important.

Or the grid can be turned landscape so that four elements are on each row.

The **second grid** is also a hierarchy, but this time it divides the elements up from the top to the bottom rows rather like Maslow's 'Hierarchy of Needs' diagram, narrowing towards the top. For this diagram there are only ten spaces.

These two diagrams can be used in conjunction with one another. First determine the twelve most important elements using the 3 × 4 grid. Then, move them to the second grid in order to determine the individual hierarchy.

This can be shared with a talk partner for the other to share their decisions and why they arrived at their unique conclusions.

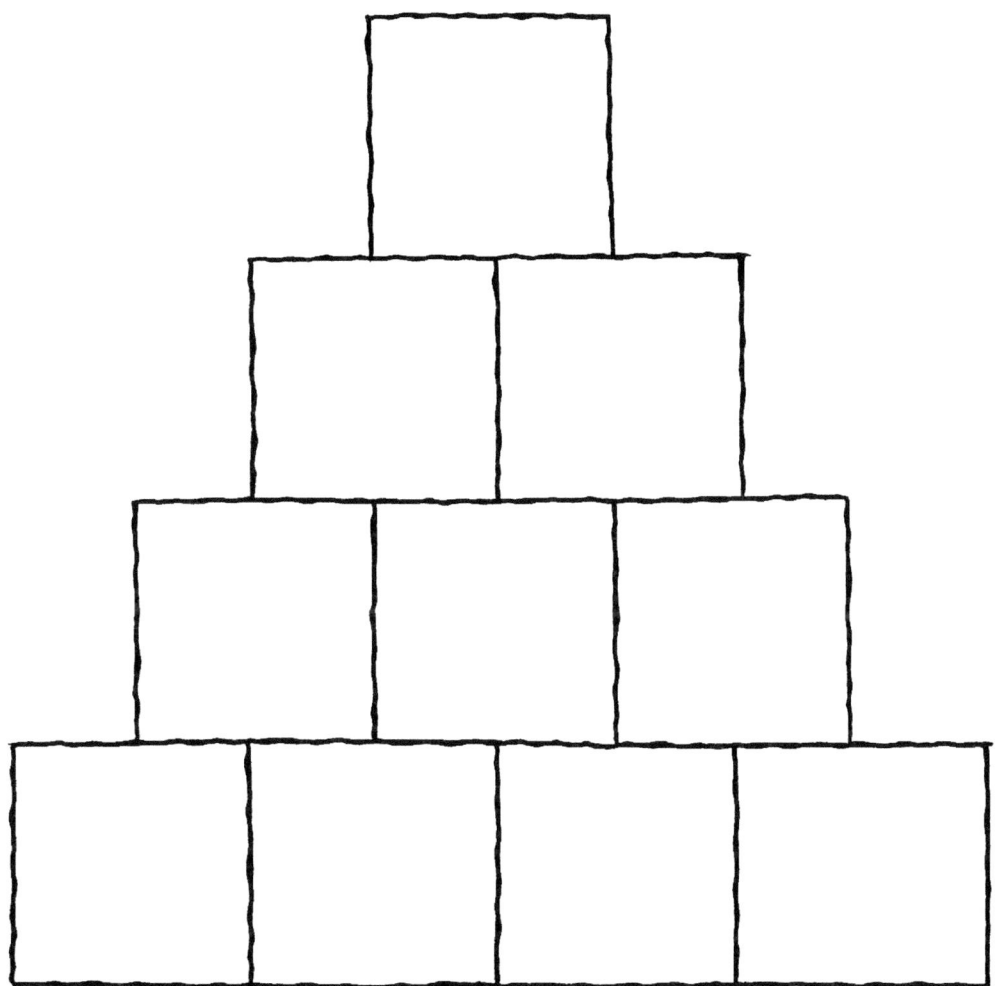

Priorities in hierarchy

CHILDREN'S HUMAN RIGHTS

Blob Human Rights Priority Cut-Out Sheet

Look at the images in the cut-out sheet with your group.

Allow pairs some time to decide what each image might represent with their talk partner. You may need to provide the list of forty-two Children's Rights Articles.

Agree as a group what the images symbolise. Some children may point out that other issues have been left out. This exercise is to prioritise the twelve images here. Some of them encompass more than one human right.

Cut up the images and provide your group with one of the two grids. Discuss how they need to use them and then provide sufficient time to first produce their own hierarchy of human rights and then secondly to discuss with their talk partner and modify their own.

A group discussion could follow to share how different people are in their priorities of human rights.

The key conclusion to draw out is that **all** forty-two of the Children's Human Rights are important and that even if we think that some are more important than others, they support the rights of everyone.

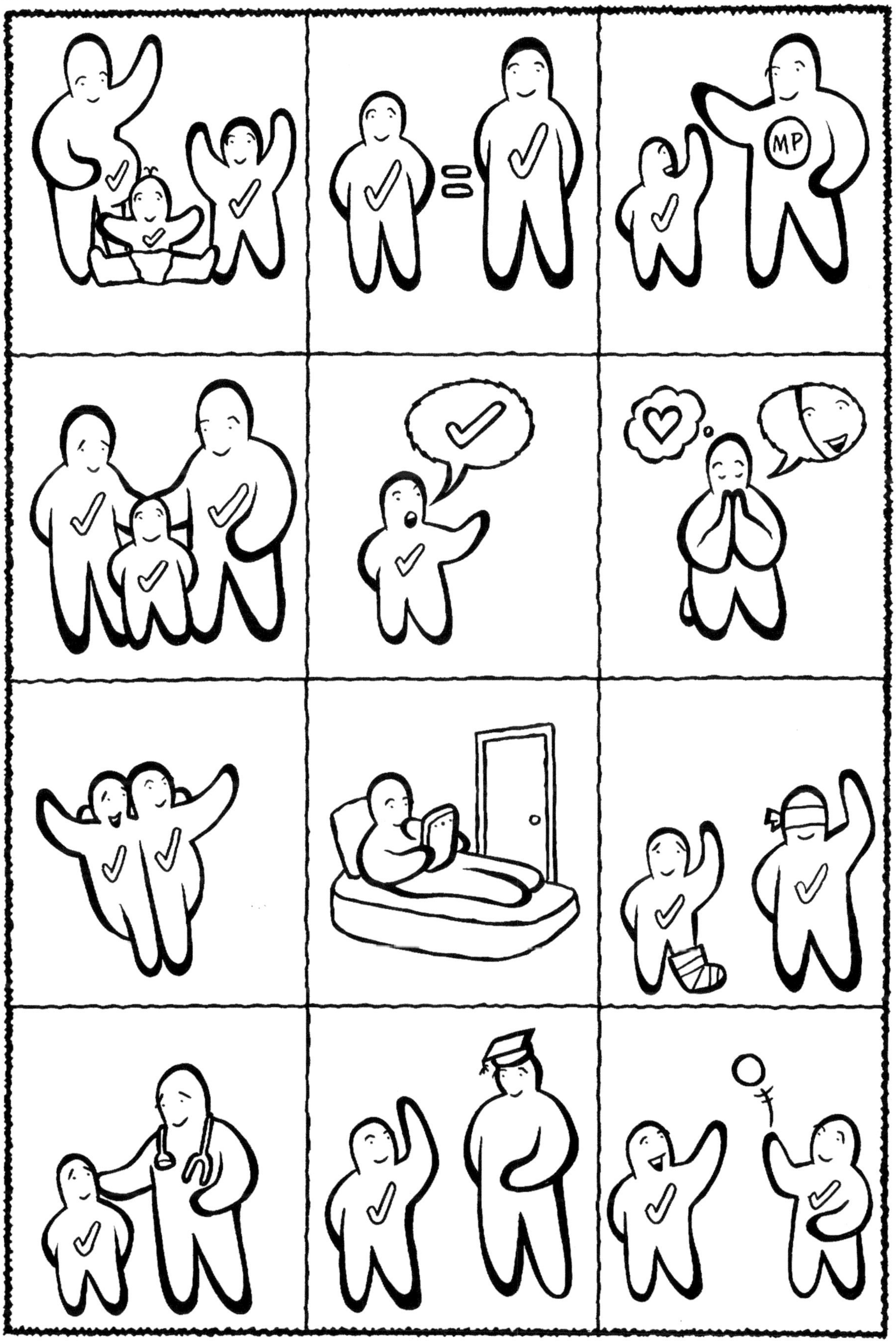

CHILDREN'S HUMAN RIGHTS

Blob Needs Priority Cut-Out Sheet

Look at the images in the cut-out sheet with your group. These are based upon the idea of essential needs.

Allow pairs some time to decide what each image might represent with their talk partner.

Agree as a group what the images symbolise. Some children may point out that other essential needs have been left out. This exercise is to prioritise the twelve images represented here.

Cut up the images and provide your group with one of the two grids. Discuss how they need to use them and then provide sufficient time to first produce their own hierarchy of human needs and then secondly to discuss with their talk partner and modify their own.

A group discussion could follow to share how different people are in their priorities of human needs.

The key conclusion to draw out is that **many of the human rights have been drawn from this list of essential needs**.

You may like to share the image of Maslow's Hierarchy of Needs to see how his compares to your group's.

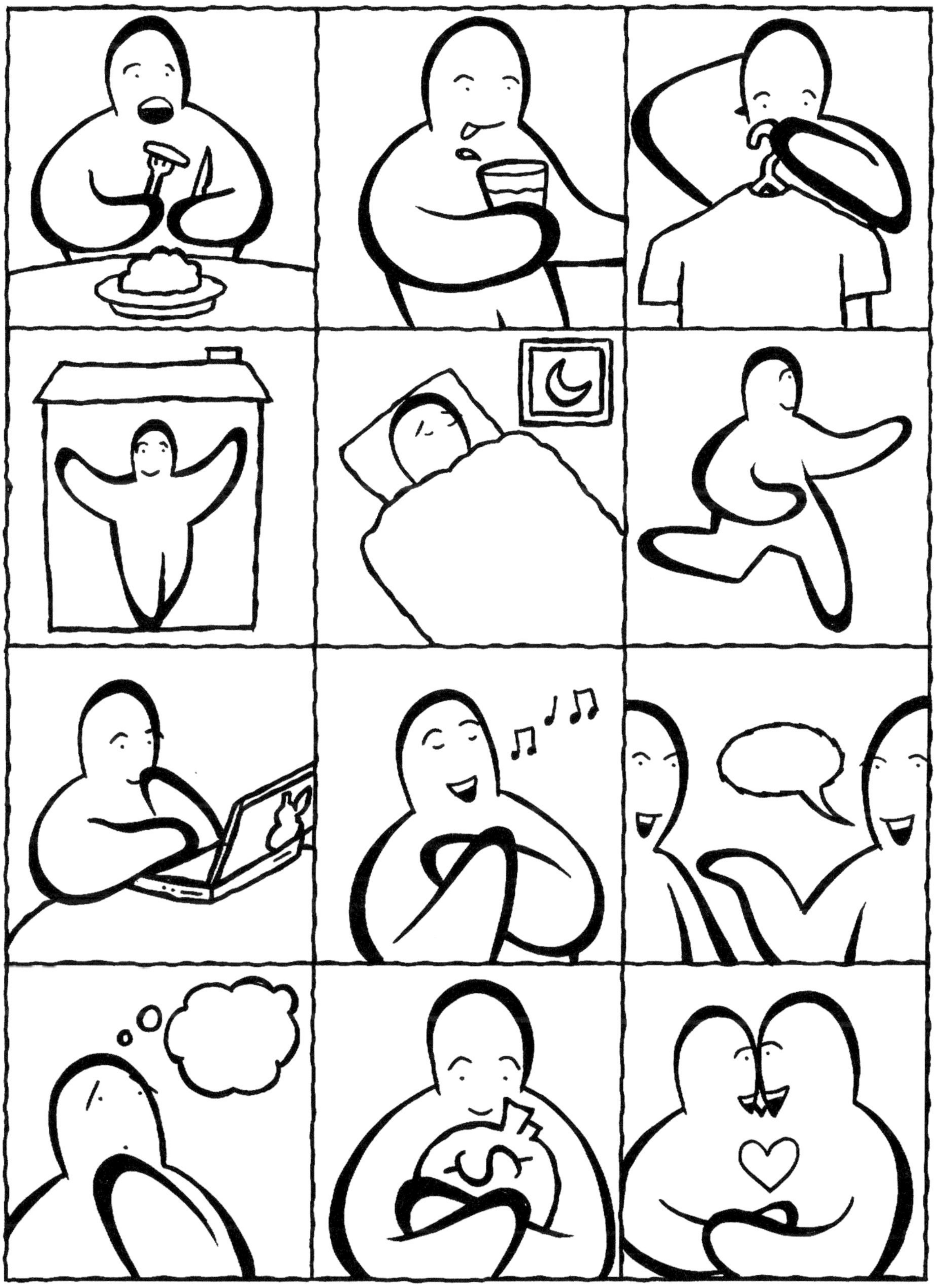

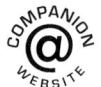

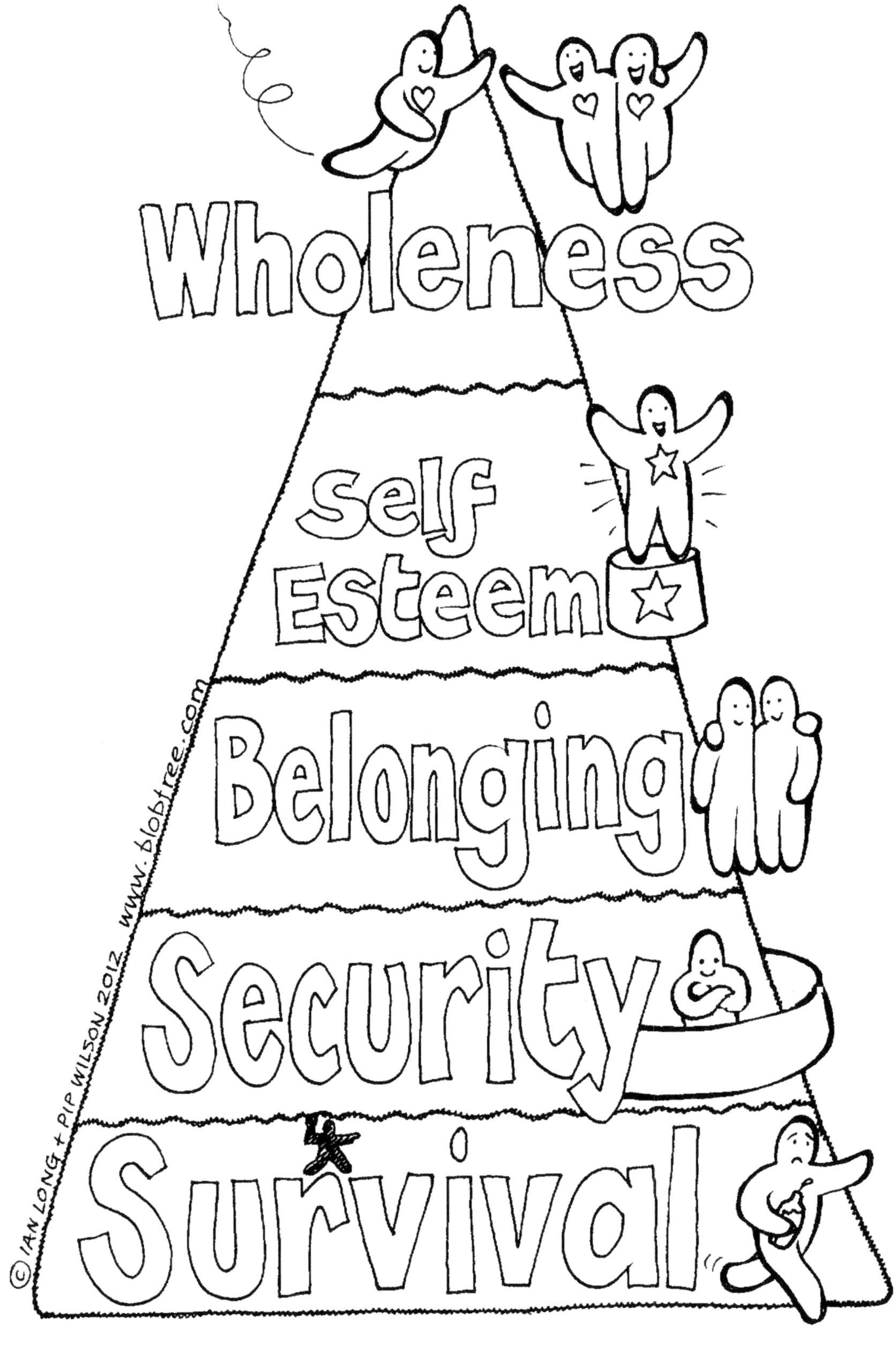

Wholeness

Self Esteem

Belonging

Security & Survival

© IAN LONG + PIP WILSON 2012 www.blobtree.com

Blob Maslow

Blob Needs and Wants Priority Cut-Out Sheet

Look at the images in the cut-out sheet with your group. These are based upon the idea of needs and wants.

Allow pairs some time to decide what each image might represent with their talk partner.

Agree as a group what the images symbolise. Some children may point out that other needs and desires have been left out. This exercise is to prioritise the twelve images represented here.

Cut up the images and provide your group with one of the two grids. Discuss how they need to use them and then provide sufficient time to first produce their own hierarchy of human needs and wants and then secondly to discuss with their talk partner and modify their own.

A group discussion could follow to share how different people are in their priorities of human needs and wants.

The key conclusion to draw out is that not all of our desires and wants are linked to human rights but many are.

You may like to share the image of Maslow's Hierarchy of Needs to see how his compares to your group's. His diagram encompasses the essential needs of the lower levels with the higher levels where aspects of creativity, self-enrichment and purpose can be found.

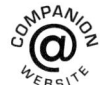

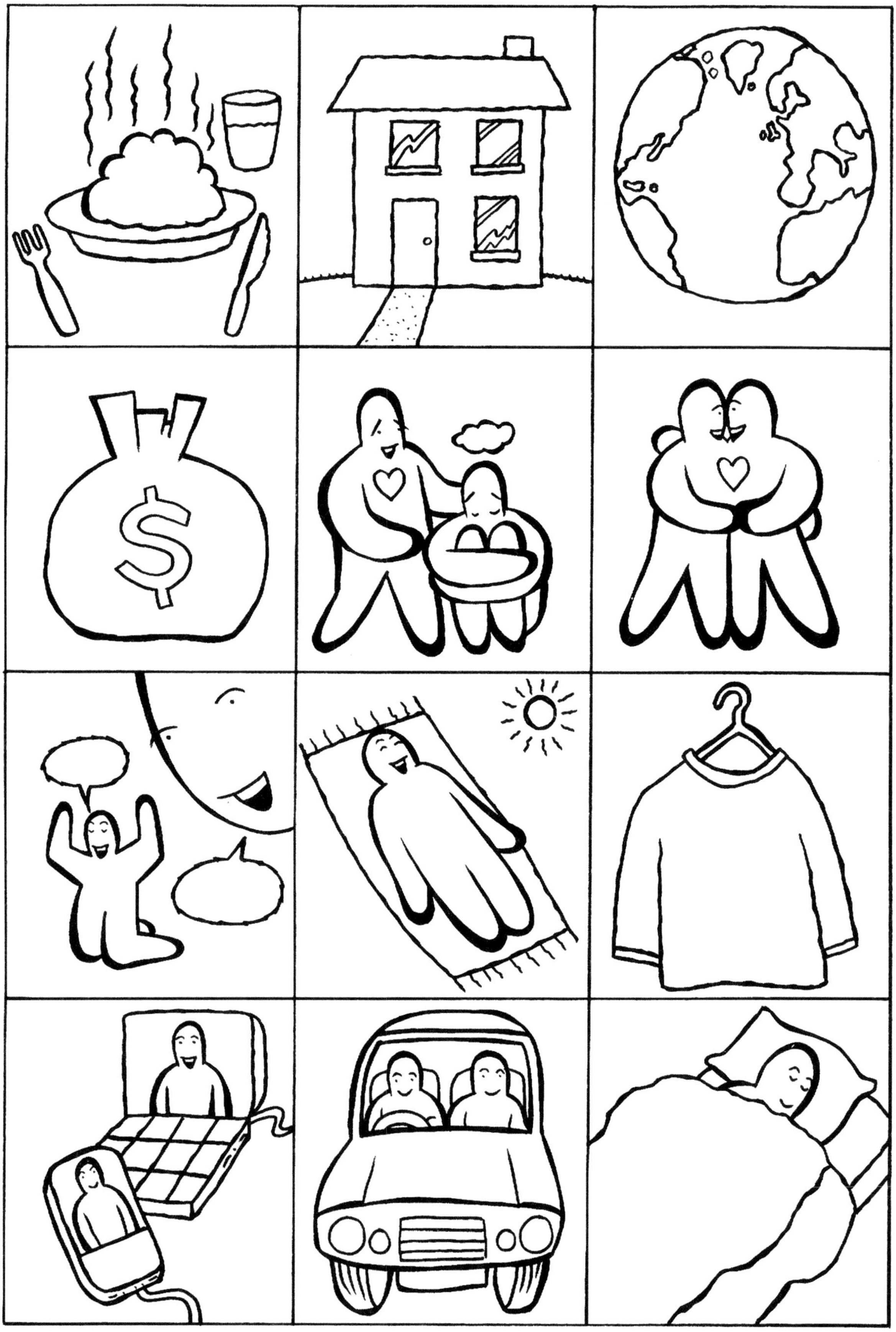

Blob
Reflective
Images

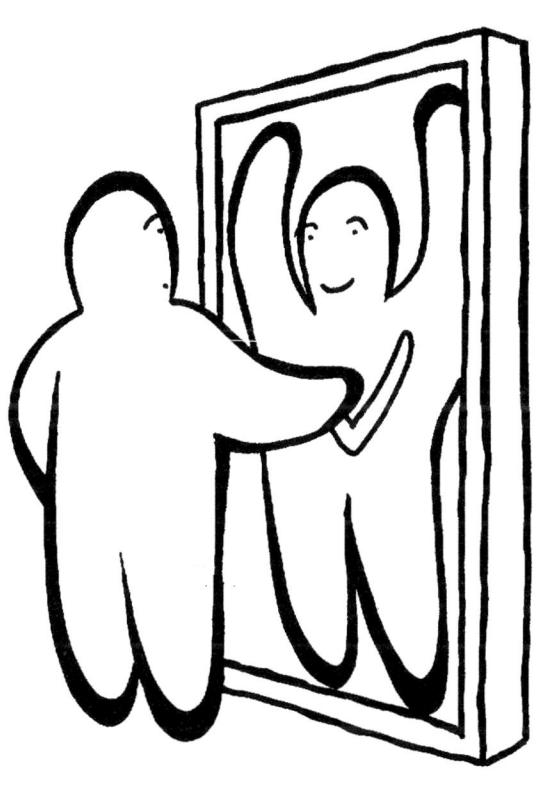

Blob Reflective Images

Human rights are important to discuss factually, but they also need to be looked at for the feelings that they create. Many children feel lonely, for example, when they can't play with their friends. When they can play with their friends, it can create a sense of belonging, being valued and wanted. The following five sheets can be used to discuss how having human rights creates a sense of safety and security.

You might like to print the images out and get the children to annotate them by passing them around small table groups.

You could project them on a whiteboard and get the children to call out appropriate feelings words whilst you or another adult write the words up.

The important outcome is for the children to realise how children's human rights create positive feelings.

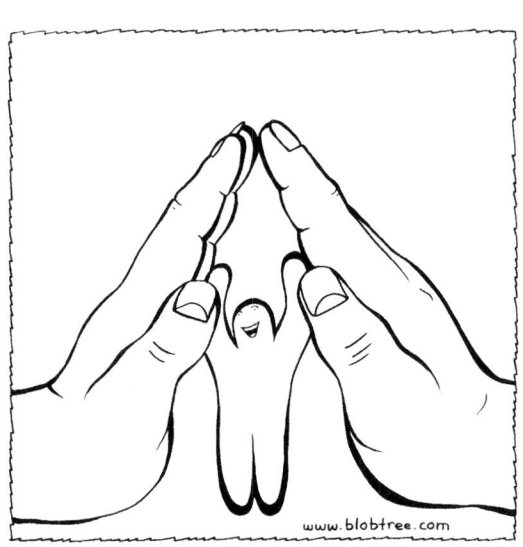

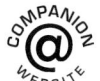

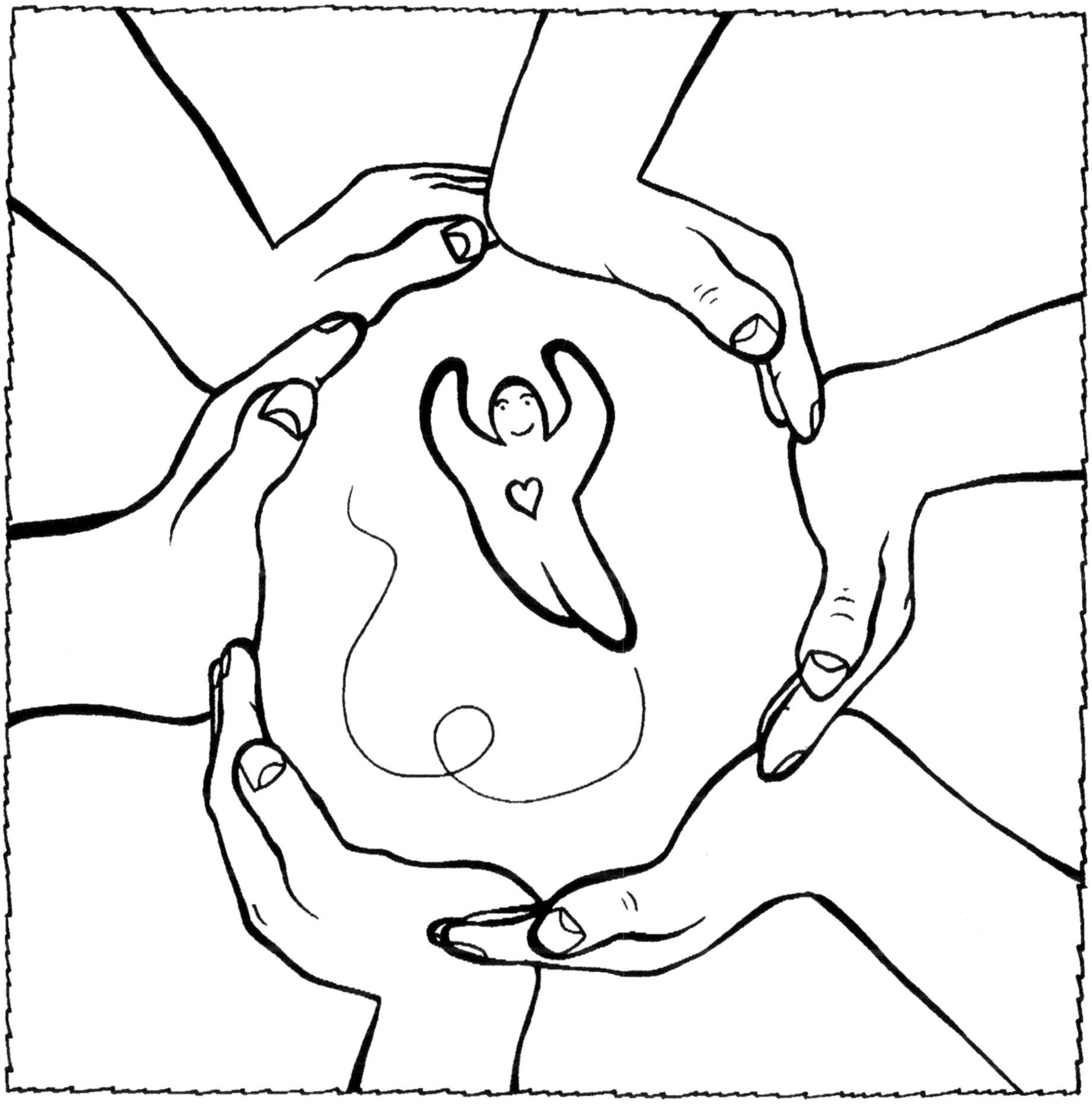

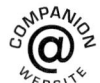

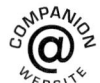

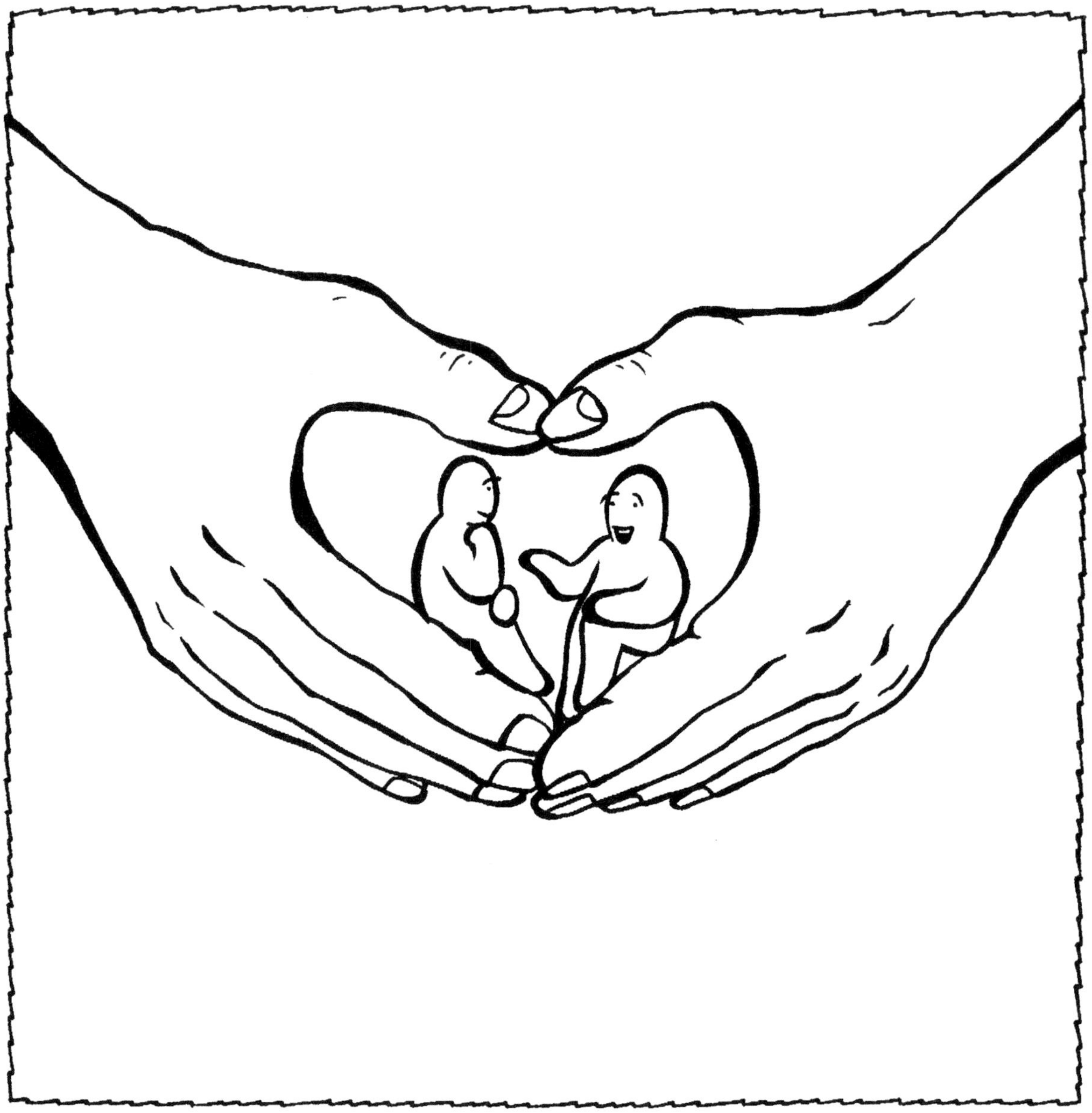

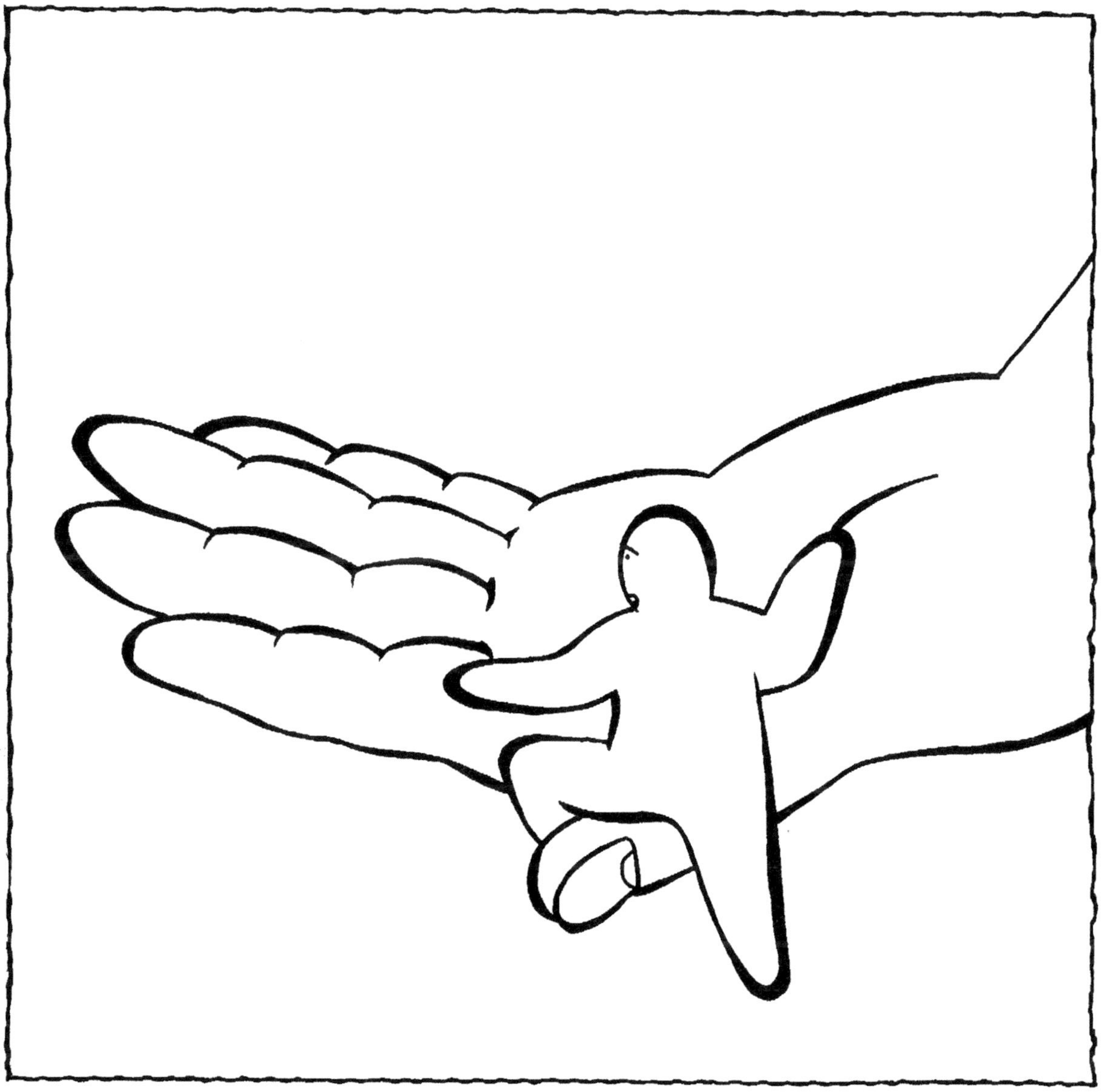

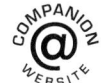

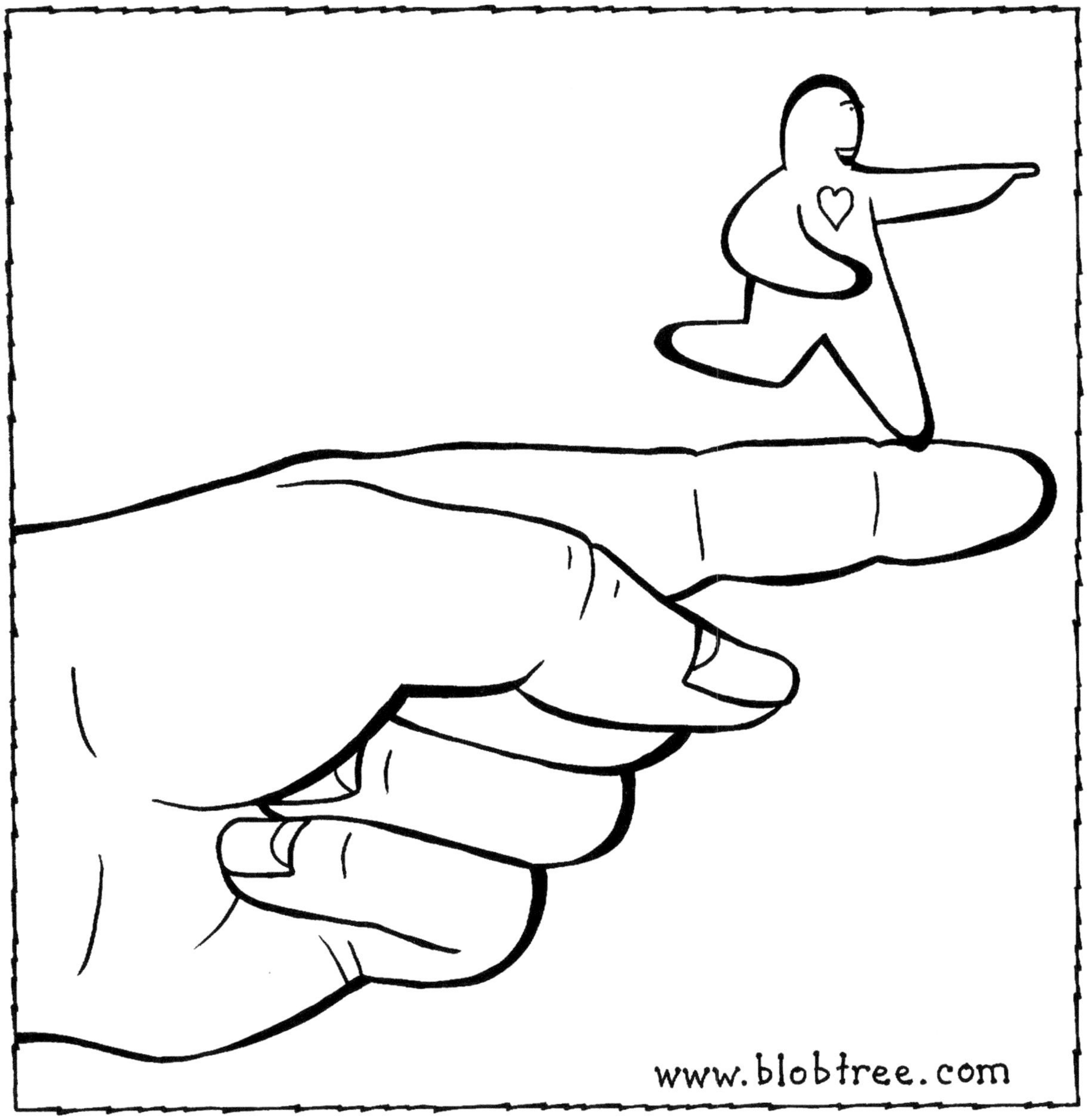

www.blobtree.com

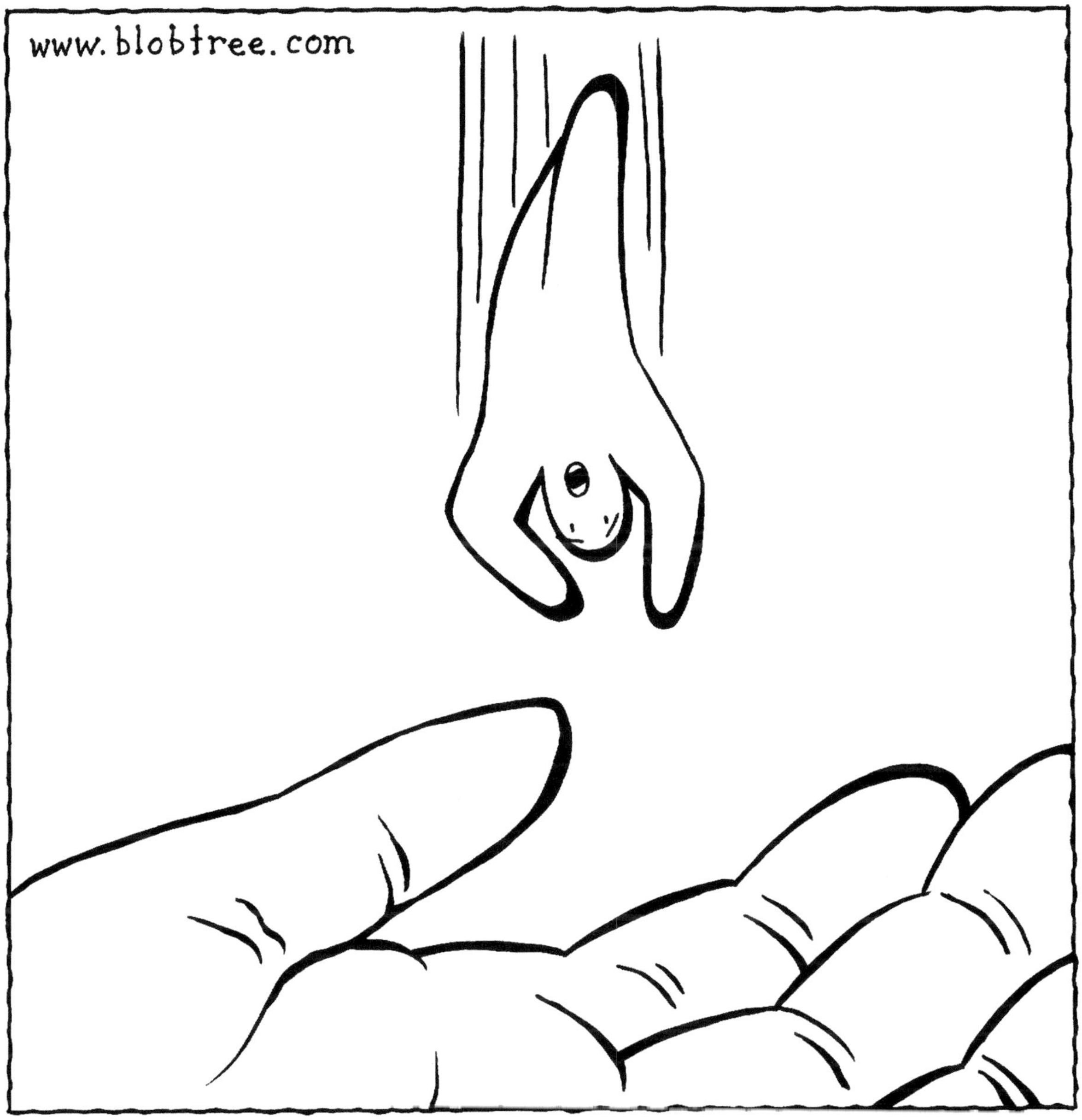

www.blobtree.com

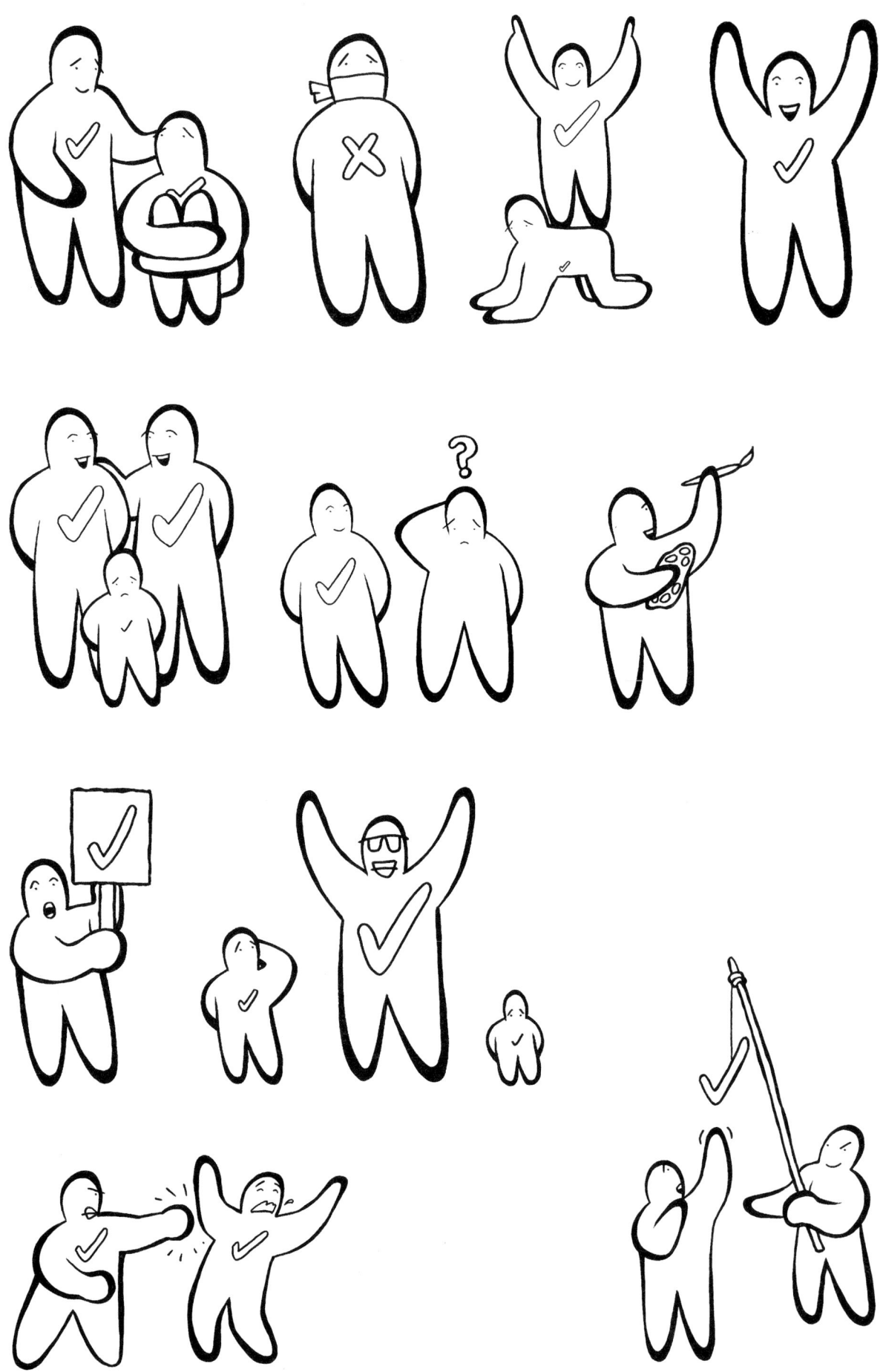